OXFORD MEDICAL PUBLICATIONS

Divine Therapy

Other works by Janet Sayers

Biological Politics:
Feminist and Anti-Feminist Perspectives

Sexual Contradictions:
Psychology, Psychoanalysis, and Feminism

Engels Revisited: New Feminist Essays
(with M. Evans and N. Redclift)

Viola Klein: The Feminine Character
(editor)

Mothering psychoanalysis: Helene Deutsch,
Karen Horney, Anna Freud, Melanie Klein

Freudian Tales or *The Man Who Never Was*

Boy Crazy: Remembering Adolescence

Kleinians: Psychoanalysis Inside Out

Divine Therapy
Love, mysticism, and psychoanalysis

Janet Sayers

OXFORD
UNIVERSITY PRESS

OXFORD
UNIVERSITY PRESS

Great Clarendon Street, Oxford OX2 6DP

Oxford University Press is a department of the University of Oxford.
It furthers the University's objective of excellence in research, scholarship,
and education by publishing worldwide in

Oxford New York

Auckland Bangkok Buenos Aires Cape Town Chennai
Dar es Salaam Hong Kong Istanbul Karachi Kolkota
Kuala Lumpur Madrid Melbourne Mexico City Mumbai
Nairobi São Paulo Shanghai Taipei Tokyo Toronto

Oxford is a registered trade mark of Oxford University Press
in the UK and in certain other countries

Published in the United States
by Oxford University Press Inc., New York

British Library Cataloguing in Publication Data

Data available

Library of Congress Cataloguing in Publication Data

Data available

ISBN 0-19-850981-2
10 9 8 7 6 5 4 3 2 1

Typeset by Newgen Imaging Systems (P) Ltd., Chennai, India
Printed in Great Britain
on acid-free paper by
Biddles Ltd, Guildford & King's Lynn

Contents

List of Illustrations

Acknowledgements

I am grateful to many people in writing this book: to my friends and family, including my Sayers, Toulson, and Brownjohn relatives for teaching me about love and about religion, negative and positive, atheist and agnostic, Christian and Jewish; to those at Dartington Hall School who first introduced me to psychoanalysis; to John Wisdom at Cambridge, who through his teaching and essay, "Gods", first taught me about relating psychoanalysis to religion; to Ronnie Laing, John Bowlby, and others at London's Tavistock Clinic from whom I first learnt about existentialism, Melanie Klein, Donald Winnicott, and Wilfred Bion; to fellow members of the British Association of Psychotherapists; to psychotherapy patients in Canterbury; and to students and fellow teachers at the University of Kent. I am also grateful to Richard Marley, at Oxford University Press, for encouraging me to write this book, to various unknown referees for their ideas about how to improve it, and to Desmond Avery without whom it would never have been written. I am also grateful to the following, in alphabetical order, for reading and commenting on one or more preliminary versions of its various chapters: Stella Ambache, Francesca Bion, Nina Farhi, Martin Golding, John Hills, Linda Hopkins, Katie Joice, Joel Kanter, Caroline New, Jan Pahl, Richard Read, Chris Ross, Hester Solomon, David Tuckett, James Williams and Roger Willoughby. Whether or not they agree, or would have agreed, with what I have written, my thanks again to the above for all they have taught me.

List of Abbreviations

BPAS   British Psycho-Analytical Society

CW   *The Collected Works of C.G. Jung*, London: Routledge & Kegan Paul, 1953–91

IJPA   *International Journal of Psycho-Analysis*

IPA   International Psycho-Analytical Association

SE   *The Standard Edition of the Complete Psychological Works of Sigmund Freud*, London: The Hogarth Press, 1955

WMK   *The Writings of Melanie Klein*, London: Hogarth, 1975

When love, with one another so
   Interinanimates two soules,
That abler soule, which thence doth flow,
   Defects lonelinesse controules.
Wee then, who are this new soule, know,
   Of what we are compos'd, and made

from *The Extasie* by John Donne

Introduction

Poets note the illuminating insights of oneness with another in love. So too do many others, including psychotherapists. But something strange and unnerving is happening. Born of love, psychotherapy is recovering it together with religion. Once wary of talking about love,[1] psychotherapists and psychoanalysts are again talking about it. Once wary of religion, indeed often downright hostile to it, they are now becomingly increasingly friendly towards it.

In telling something of how this has come about, *Divine Therapy* tells a love story, or collection of love stories to dip into as you will. Together they recount the love inspiring those contributing to making therapy what it is today. In telling their stories I will quote extensively from love letters. I will also draw on other details of their lives. Most of all I will dwell on these contributors' published writing about love, psychology, mysticism, and religion.

In doing all this I will draw more on men's than on women's writing, such is the continuing effect of men's social dominance, both now and in the past. Also symptomatic of this dominance is my using "he", "his", "him", and other male words to stand, generically, for both sexes whenever I cannot find a way of avoiding cumbersome non-sexist language. Like those whose work I recount, I will also talk about "health" and "illness", and about "doctors" and "patients", thereby reflecting the continuing medicalization of the spiritual and psychological distress for which people seek help, despite reservations, as I will indicate in due course, raised long ago against this practice by several of those with whose work I deal.

There are good reasons not to medicalize women's and men's unhappiness. There are also good reasons not to equate psychoanalysis with psychotherapy or with religion. Nevertheless I will do so in certain respects – indeed it is one of my major aims in this book to bring all three together. Above all I aim to demonstrate that, like religion, psychoanalysis and psychotherapy seek to animate or reanimate the psyche or soul of their recipients through the medium of the psychoanalyst's or psychotherapist's oneness with his or her patients. This entails the oneness that lies at the heart of mystical and religious experience, and also at the heart of falling in love, making love, and being in love. For many it may involve experiencing oneness with God or with another as divine.

----

[1] Hester McFarland Solomon (1998) Love: Paradox of self and other, in D. Mann (2002) *Love and Hate: Psychoanalytic Perspectives*, London: Brunner Routledge, pp. 53–67.

But this, of course, is a contradiction. It is, at best, a fiction to imagine oneself to be one with another, mortal or immortal, finite or infinite, personal or impersonal, human or divine. So struck was Freud by this contradiction that he dismissed it as an illusion. He diagnosed it as a defensive retreat to what he variously called "the oceanic feeling" or "primary narcissism" of earliest infancy. One of his first and most influential followers, Karl Abraham, described it as the essence of manic grandiosity and paradoxically, as also the essence of melancholic despair. Abraham's analysand and colleague, Melanie Klein, described it as regression to a "phantasy" of "projective identification" characteristic, she said, of our developmentally earliest "paranoid–schizoid" state of mind.

Long before these psychoanalysts thus questioned the oneness with another which many writers over the centuries have equated with love and with religious experience, the philosopher Hegel deplored this implied conflation of love with religion. Writing at the height of the early nineteenth century Romantic revolution in European art and literature, he complained that "this secular religion of the heart", as he described love, "now unites itself with religion every way". True to his philosophy of dialectics, he wrote of the contradictions of love. He drew attention to the fact that love's aims, as he put it, "cannot be achieved in a concrete reality without collisions, because the other relations of life assert their demands and rights".[2]

In being about love, as well as about religion, this book is also about what Hegel called love's collisions. They are graphically evoked by Epstein's statue, *Jacob and the Angel*, in London's Tate Britain Gallery. A note beside it explains:

> Jacob, the Old Testament patriarch whose twelve sons founded the twelve tribes of Israel, was a central figure in Judaism. The Book of Genesis describes a mysterious crisis in his life, when he wrestled all night with a divine stranger, an angel, whom he almost overcame . . . The angel of the Bible story was able to restrain Jacob only by dislocating his hip, and the moment portrayed seems to be just after that, with the angel supporting Jacob who has collapsed. This was the moment when Jacob understood that he had been fighting against God.

So much do fighting and collisions with God, and also with love, bruise and batter us, that many say we are better off without them. Of love, one might cynically ask, like the television comic Lily Tomlin, "If love is the answer, could you rephrase the question?" Love's collisions might tempt us to dismiss it, as some feminists do, as nothing but a snare and delusion, a mystifying source of women's (and men's) complicity in their oppression.

One might say the same of religion. Just as considerable damage has been done in the name of love, so too considerable damage has been done in the

---

[2] G.W.F. Hegel (1835) *Aesthetics*, Vol. I, Oxford: Clarendon Press, 1975, p. 565.

name of religion. At best, it is said, religion is a sop. It is an opium of the people. Thank goodness, say some, that (as the philosopher Friedrich Nietzsche is often quoted as saying) "God is dead". But is God dead? Is religion – theistic or non-theistic – gone? Not at all. It still wrecks havoc and does dreadful harm. Its effects can be cataclysmic. But it can also be a force for good. Islam and other religions remain a major source of inspiration, across the world, of women's and men's struggles for freedom.

Far from being dead, religion is alive and well. There is also mounting evidence that religion is good for our physical and mental well-being. So considerable is this evidence that it has persuaded researchers working for the World Health Organization in Geneva to seek ways of refining items assessing women's and men's spiritual, religious, and personal belief to measure its correlation with measures of their overall quality of life.[3] But is religion – or holiness – good for our quality of life, well-being, and physical or mental health? And if it is, what are the implications for therapy?

It was with this last question that I originally began. In seeking answers I returned to lectures given in Edinburgh in 1901 and in 1902 by the Harvard psychologist, William James, brother of the more famous novelist, Henry James. In Chapter 1, I recount how William James' love of his father, wife, and later of a young woman, Pauline Goldmark, as well as other biographical factors contributed to his arguing in his Edinburgh lectures that religion can heal what he described as "the divided self" of "the sick soul" through love of, and oneness with, the goodness of God mediated through the unconscious.

This takes me to Freud's discoveries about the unconscious. Arguably these were inspired in large part by Freud's love of a fellow-doctor, Wilhelm Fliess. Recounting this in Chapter 2, I also recount Freud's discoveries of means of accessing the unconscious through what he described as "free association" and through the "transference-love" and defences against love evoked in patients by their doctors and psychoanalysts. In detailing this I also detail Freud's rejection of religion and religious or mystical experience as contrary to the scientific pursuit of truth by psychoanalysis, not least the truth of sex and love.

Jung, by contrast, was much more friendly to religion. As I explain in Chapter 3, he was also more friendly than Freud to the healing effects of counter-transference feelings evoked in doctors and psychoanalysts by their patients. In this, I will argue, Jung was inspired by the love of one of his patients, Sabina Spielrein. Ironically, however, although Jung emphasized the

---

[3] The World Health Organization's quality of life project into spirituality, religiousness and personal beliefs, unpublished report, presented by S. Skevington and K. O'Connell in Geneva in February 2000.

beneficial effects of the mutual influences of patients and their doctors or psychoanalysts on each other in bringing about their healing oneness with God and other archetypes, as he put it, in the collective unconscious, Jung lost sight of the dyadic – I/Thou – character of women's and men's relation to God. Like William James, Jung emphasized the therapeutic effect of oneness with God; but whereas James said that this oneness is mediated *by* the unconscious, Jung argued that it involves oneness with God *in* the unconscious.

This is to go against the tenets of all established religion and mystical experience. The dyadic character of this experience is particularly well brought out in the religious and autobiographical writing of the political theorist and activist, Simone Weil, to whom I turn in Chapter 4. Through her writing, she eloquently and movingly highlights recovery from self-alienation through mystical experiences of oneness with God. In doing so, as I will explain, she equated God with what Plato called goodness, and thereby very much emphasized the dyadic character of religious experience as a relation, oriented by what she called the light of love, to what is entirely outside, prior to, and beyond us.

Jung's version of religion and psychoanalysis not only overlooks this dyadic character of religious experience but is also authoritarian – or at least that is what the sociologist and psychoanalyst, Erich Fromm argued influentially, as I explain in Chapter 5. In doing so I also outline Fromm's alternative, humanist version of religion and psychoanalysis, as well as the parallels he draws between psychoanalysis and Buddhism as means of achieving spiritual enlightenment.

Ironically however, Fromm, like Jung, also tended to lose sight of the dyadic character of religious experience. Arguably he developed an overly individualistic version of psychoanalysis and religion. Fromm's New York colleague, Paul Tillich, whose existentialist account of religion and psychoanalysis was particularly influential, chided him for this. In Chapter 6, I explain Tillich's theory and recount his theory of the healing of self-division through grace involving accepting being accepted by another recognized as separate and different in being infinite, immortal, and divine.

I then illustrate, in Chapter 7, the application to therapy of the philosophy of existentialism, pioneered by Heidegger and developed by Tillich, as further developed by the Viennese psychiatrist Viktor Frankl. I describe how, in forging what he called "logotherapy" from religion and psychoanalysis, Frankl was inspired by his own spiritual transformation from soulless meaninglessness through recalling his love of his wife, Tilly, when they were both imprisoned in concentration camps during the Second World War.

Frankl, however, was arguably over-optimistic in his approach to therapy. Certainly he emphasized love and said little about hate. Not so Melanie Klein.

She very much emphasized both in her account of psychoanalysis as means of transforming self-division and self-fragmentation through oneness with another internalized as loving, loved, and good. She drew parallels between this and Christian rites and rituals. But, as I also document in Chapter 8, she was generally hostile to religion, both in her early work in pioneering child analysis, and in her later secular account of the transformations wrought by psychoanalysis, in which she tended to focus more on inner than on outer reality. This imbalance, however, was very much put to rights by her follower, the art critic, Adrian Stokes, with whose work I accordingly end this chapter.

Adrian Stokes emphasized healing oneness with what he called the "object–otherness" of art. This takes me to the work of the artist and psychoanalyst, Marion Milner. Like Stokes, she too emphasized the healing effect of marrying inwardness with outwardness. In this, as I illustrate with many examples in Chapter 9, she drew on insights acquired through experiments with mysticism which she applied in her own self-analysis, in her work in child analysis, and in incorporating art therapy into her psychoanalytic work with adults. In doing so she emphasized the healing effect of recovering the illusion of oneness with another involved in being in love and in religious or mystical experience, previously dismissed by psychoanalysts (as indicated above) as a defensive retreat to childhood ways of feeling and thinking.

But where does the illusion of oneness with another, and where do our illusions and dreams generally first come from? This brings me to the work of the psychoanalyst and paediatrician, Donald Winnicott, and to his account of our illusions first being inspired, or at least fuelled, through our mothers' oneness with us as babies enabling our mothers to imagine and thereby feed our illusions with details of what is actually there. This in turn, said Winnicott, fosters the development of what he described as "a transitional space", in which we begin to recognize ourselves as both one with, and separate from others and the world around us. This is also the space, Winnicott wrote, of "religious feeling".

Winnicott was not particularly religious. Nor was the psychiatrist and psychoanalyst, Wilfred Bion, whose work I seek to explain in Chapter 11. Like Winnicott, however, Bion also emphasized the oneness of psychoanalysts with their patients as main means of transforming their soul or psyche, as one could put it, from thing-like deadness to spiritual aliveness. Bion likened this oneness to what he called the mystic's "at-one-ment" with "ultimate reality" or "O". He arrived at this theory through insights about treating patients suffering with psychosis. These insights themselves, I will argue, were initially inspired by Bion's love of a young woman, Francesca, who became his wife.

True to the wariness of psychoanalysts about talking about love, few of the above-mentioned psychoanalysts say much about it in their published writing about psychoanalysis and religion. The leading feminist and literary theorist, Julia Kristeva, however, says a great deal about love. She is one of the most prominent people currently resurrecting love, within psychoanalysis, in association with religion. She insists that the love of psychoanalysts for their patients, akin to Christ's injunction to love one's neighbour as oneself, is central to the oneness through which, she says, the analyst gives semiotic meaning to the patient's symptoms. The psychoanalyst, she says, thereby heals the phobias, psychoses, melancholia, soul sickness, pathological guilt, anorexia, or autism that can result from experiencing oneself not as spiritually alive but as driven by a meaningless instinct, drive, will, or thing. Kristeva likens the transformation achieved in psychoanalysis through love to the transubstantiation of the body and blood of Christ into bread and wine in Holy Communion, and to the iconography of the Madonna and infant Christ of the Russian Orthodox religion in which she first grew up in Bulgaria.

Kristeva's account of love, religion, and psychoanalysis, which I seek to explain in Chapter 12, brings me to the conclusion of my book. Now, having outlined in very condensed form its contents, I will expand them in much greater detail, starting with the life and work of William James who, as I will seek to demonstrate in subsequent chapters, laid the groundwork of what is best in today's integration of psychotherapy with psychoanalysis, mysticism, and religion.

Chapter 1

William James

Divided self

William James was one of the foremost founders of current research into the psychology of religion. As I have indicated, he also laid out many of the major themes – not least concerning free will (psyche or spirit) and its divisions – taken up subsequently by psychologists, doctors, and others in relating religion, therapy, and mental health. James valued religious experience for its therapeutic and generally beneficial practical effects. In so doing he sidelined the issue of whether belief in God is true, whatever its practical or therapeutic benefits. By focusing on individual religious experience, James overlooked its interpersonal, communal, social, cross-cultural, and historical determinants. He also overlooked the cultural determinants of his own individualistic perspective on religion.

Nevertheless his work is also immensely appealing and is both evocative and inspiring in the way it relates religious experience to what is most ineffable and inspiring in love. His personal warmth and sympathy with others also makes his writing a pleasure to read. Many say he was a better writer, though perhaps not as good a psychologist, as his novelist brother, Henry. Certainly I find his writing illuminating. In quoting it, I will also dwell on factors in William James' personal life – particularly his experience of self-division – that contributed to his final account of religious experience as therapy. I will begin, however, with his boyhood and youth.

Divided youth

William James was born in New York on 11 January 1842. He was the oldest of five children.[1] Undecided as to what would be best for them in terms of their upbringing and education, their father sent them to diverse educational institutions. He also employed various governesses and tutors for them in their successive homes in Albany, in upstate New York, Manhattan, London, Geneva,

---

[1] William's brothers and sister, in order of age, were Henry (born on 15 April 1843), Garth Wilkinson (born on 21 July 1845), Robertson (born in August 1846), and Alice (born on 7 August 1848).

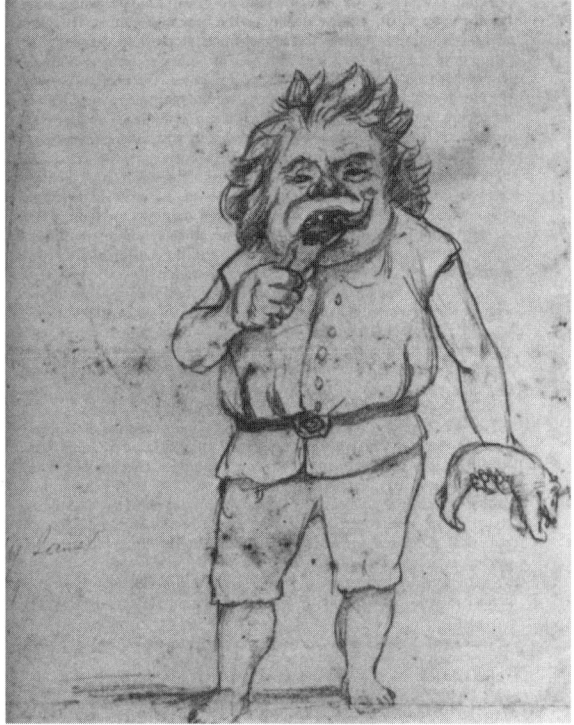

Fig. 1.1 Drawing of a Giant – by William James.

Paris, Boulogne, Bonn, and in Newport, Rhode Island, where they finally settled. Recalling their itinerant youth, William's slightly younger brother, Henry, later wrote: "we were never faithful long, or for more than one winter, to the same studious scene".[2] He also recalled William from their Manhattan days:

> As I catch W.J.'s image, from far back, at its most characteristic, he sits drawing and drawing, always drawing, especially under the lamplight of the Fourteenth Street back parlour; and not as with a plodding patience, which I think would less have affected me, but easily, freely and, as who should say, infallibly: always at the stage of finishing off, his head dropped from side to side and his tongue rubbing his lower lip.[3]

In contrast, what William remembered from this time was his father's coldness and iron discipline: "I never suffered more pain", he later wrote to his sister, "since Father used to spank me with a paper cutter in fourteenth street".[4] When he was young he drew a picture (Fig. 1.1), arguably based on his fraught relationship

---

[2] H. James (1913, 1914, 1917) *Autobiography*, London: W. H. Allen, 1956 p. 14.

[3] Ibid. p. 118.

[4] To Alice James, 31 August 1865, in L. Simon (1998) *Genuine Reality: A Life of William James*, New York: Harcourt Brace, p. 40.

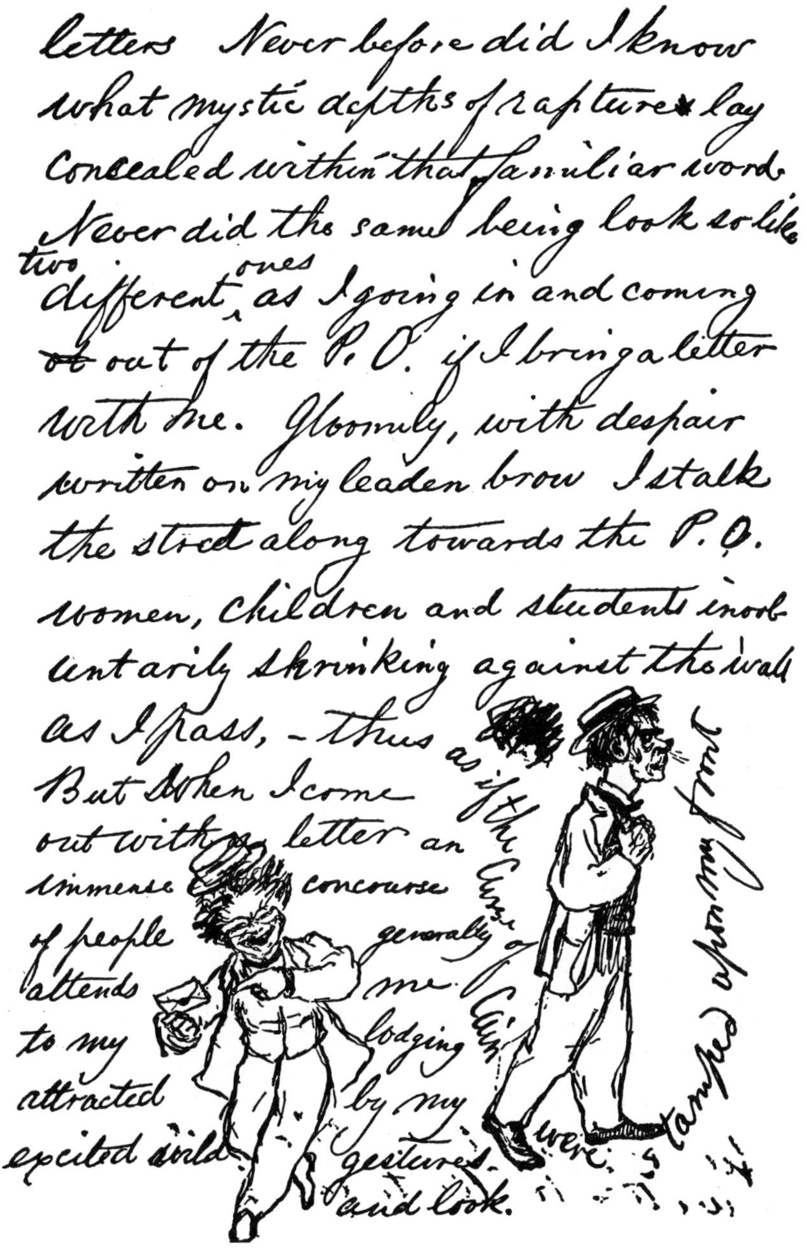

letters Never before did I know
what mystic depths of rapture* lay
concealed within that familiar word.
Never did the same being look so like
two different ones as I going in and coming
~~ot~~ out of the P.O. if I bring a letter
with me. Gloomily, with despair
written on my leaden brow I stalk
the street along towards the P.O.
women, children and students invol-
untarily shrinking against the wall
as I pass, — thus as if the curse of Cain were stamped upon my front
But when I come
out with a letter an
immense concourse
of people generally
attends me
to my lodging
attracted by my
excited wild gestures
and look.

Fig. 1.2 Letter from William James to his family.

with his father, of a man-eating ogre.[5] The divisions between them became increasingly bitter when William's father sent him to Bonn to learn German in order to prepare him to study science in Frankfurt. Their divisions, however, were resolved by William's father conceding to William's wish to study painting with William Morris Hunt and his pupil, John La Farge, in Newport, and that September, 1860, the family returned there.

Within six months, however, William had changed his mind. Feeling he could never excel as an artist, said his brother, Henry, his "interest in the practice of painting . . . suddenly and abruptly ceased".[6] William then persuaded his father to allow him to study chemistry at Harvard – perhaps by threatening to join the army to fight in the US Civil War, which was just beginning – and wrote home from there (see Fig. 1.2), depicting in pictures and words his divided state of mind.

> Never did the same being look so like two different ones, as I going in and coming out of the P.O. if I bring a letter with me. Gloomily, with despair written on my leaden brow I stalk the street along towards the P.O. women, children and students involuntarily shrinking against the wall as I pass, – thus as if the curse of Cain were stamped upon my front. But when I come out with a letter an immense concourse of people generally attends me to my lodging attracted by my excited wild gestures and look.[7]

Many years later, William's chemistry teacher, Charles Eliot, described his indecisiveness as a student: his being "not wholly devoted to the study of Chemistry"; his work often being "interfered with by ill-health, or rather by something which I imagined to be a delicacy of nervous constitution"; his frequent "excursions into other sciences and realms of thought"; his "unusual mental powers, remarkable spirituality, and great personal charm".[8] Attracted to the teaching of the Swiss naturalist, Louis Agassiz, James began shifting his interests from chemistry to biology.

In September 1863 he wrote to his cousin, Kitty Temple (one of four orphans, whose portrait he painted, see Fig. 1.3),[9] of his indecision about his future career:

> I am obliged before the 15 January [1864] to make finally and irrevocably "the choice of a profession". I suppose your sex . . . has no idea of the awful responsibility of such a choice. I have four alternatives: Natural History, Medicine, Printing, Beggary. . . . Of all departments of Medicine, that to which Dr Prince [to whom Kitty was married] devotes himself is, I should think, the most interesting.[10]

[5] H. Feinstein (1984) *Becoming William James*, Ithaca: Cornell University Press, p. 127.

[6] H. James *Autobiography*, p. 300.

[7] From Cambridge, September 1861, in H. James p. 314.

[8] In H. James (1920a) *The Letters of William James*, London: Longmans, Green, p. 31–2.

[9] H. James, *Autobiography*, opposite, p. 293.

[10] Letter to Mrs William H. Prince, 12 September 1863, ibid. p. 43–4.

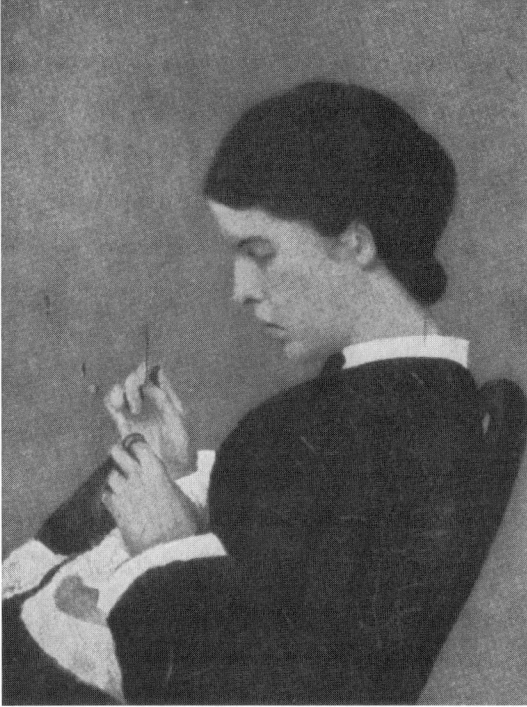

Fig. 1.3 Portrait of Katherine Temple – by William James.

The next spring, 1864, William's family joined him in Boston, and in the autumn he registered as a medical student at Harvard. He now became fearful of going mad. He worried lest coming into contact with "live lunatics", through studying psychiatry, result in his catching "their contagion", especially since he found his reason shaken by the symptoms described in a psychiatry textbook he read.[11]

Again he changed his mind about what to study. In April 1865 he joined an evolutionary biology expedition led by Agassiz to the Amazon. On arriving in Rio de Janeiro, however, William became seriously ill with a form of smallpox which temporarily stopped him seeing or reading. It also left him feeling weak and exhausted, and with a legacy of depression with which he suffered, intermittently, throughout his life. The expedition also convinced him that he was not suited to becoming a naturalist: "If there is one thing I hate", he wrote to his father, "it is collecting",[12] adding "I am convinced now for good that I am cut out for a speculative rather than an active life".[13]

[11] To Kitty Price, 13 December 1863, in Feinstein p. 304.

[12] In M. Knight (1950) *William James*, Harmondsworth: Penguin, p. 21.

[13] To Henry James Sr, 3 June 1865, in James 1920a p. 62.

On returning to Boston the following March, in 1866, he resumed his medical studies. He worked that summer as an intern in the Massachusetts General Hospital but soon had to give up the work because of back trouble. It was arguably modelled on the back trouble of his *alter ego* brother, Henry, contracted in 1861, possibly as means of getting out of fighting in the US Civil War.[14] As well as back trouble William also suffered with depression. Perhaps this was exacerbated by one of his friends, Fanny Dixwell, to whom he was attached, becoming involved with his friend, Oliver Wendell Holmes Jr.

William again quit his studies at Harvard, this time ostensibly to study physiology in Germany, but also, as he put it, to "fly from a home which had become loathsome".[15] From Europe he wrote about his bad back and suicidal thoughts. He went to a spa – Bad-Teplitz in Bohemia. But he found it made him feel as if his brain "had been boiled".[16]

Perhaps, he thought, the answer lay in free will as an alternative to religion:

> The thought that with me outlasts all others, and onto which, like a rock, I find myself washed up when the waves of doubt are weltering over all the rest of the world . . . is the thought of having a will . . . if we have to give up all hope of seeing into the purposes of God, or to give up theoretically the idea of final causes, and of God anyhow as vain and leading to nothing for us, we can, by our will, make the enjoyment of our brothers stand us in the stead of a final cause . . . The idea, in short, of becoming an accomplice in a sort of "Mankind its own God or Providence" scheme is a *practical* one.[17]

He told his sister, also faced with depression, to exert her will against it, to "keep a stiff upper lip & snap your fingers at fate".[18] But he himself remained depressed. From another spa – this time in Divonne – he wrote "I am poisoned with Utilitarian venom, and sometimes when I despair of ever doing anything, ask myself 'Why not step out into the green darkness?'"[19]

The next month, November 1868, he returned to Boston where he had blistering and electric shock treatment for his back, and in June 1869 he graduated as a doctor. The same month his cousin Kitty's younger sister, Minny,[20] was

---

[14] Knight p. 23.

[15] To Tom Ward, 12 September 1867, in Feinstein p. 207.

[16] See James 1920a p. 85.

[17] To Tom Ward from Berlin, January 1868, in James 1920a pp. 130, 132.

[18] To Alice James, 4 June 1868, in Simon p. 243.

[19] To Tom Ward from Divonne, 9 October 1868, in R. B. Perry (1935a) *The Thought and Character of William James, Vol. I*, Boston: Little, Brown, p. 287.

[20] Apparently Isabel Archer in *The Portrait of a Lady*, and Molly Teale in *The Wings of the Dove*, were both modelled on Minny, see James 1920a p. 36.

diagnosed with symptoms of TB. Perhaps this contributed to William again becoming depressed. Early the next year he wrote in his diary, "Today I about touched bottom". He was becoming suffused, he said, with what he called "the evil that seems inherent" in the universe.[21] Minny died the next month, March 1870, and soon after William wrote dejectedly in his diary about the "immediacy of death" and about "the nothingness of all our egoistic fury".[22]

He again sought the answer in free will:

> I think that yesterday was a crisis in my life. I finished the first part of Renouvier's second "Essais" and see no reason why his definition of Free Will – "the sustaining of a thought *because I choose to* when I might have other thoughts" – need be the definition of an illusion. At any rate, I will assume for the present – until next year – that it is no illusion. My first act of free will shall be to believe in free will. For the remainder of the year, I will abstain from the mere speculation and contemplative *Grüblei* [grubbing among subtleties] in which my nature takes most delight, and voluntarily cultivate the feeling of moral freedom, by reading books favorable to it, as well as by acting. . . . Hitherto, when I have felt like taking a free initiative, like daring to act originally, without carefully waiting for contemplation of the external world to determine all for me, suicide seemed the most manly form to put my daring into; now, I will go a step further with my will, not only act with it, but believe as well; believe in my individual reality and creative power. My belief, to be sure, *can't* be optimistic – but I will posit life (the real, the good) in the self-governing *resistance* of the ego to the world. Life shall [be built in] doing and suffering and creating.[23]

He wrote to his brother, Henry, of similarly resisting evil:

> It seems to me that all a man has to depend on in this world, is, in the last resort, mere brute power of resistance. I can't bring myself, as so many men seem able to, to blink the evil out of sight, and gloss it over. It's as real as the good, and if it is denied, good must be denied too. It must be accepted and hated, and resisted while there's breath in our bodies.[24]

But he remained depressed. He headed a drawing (see Fig. 1.4) with what has been described as a Freudian slip reference to his MD medical qualification, "HERE I AMD SORROW SIT".[25] Little is known of his movements between 1870 and 1872. It is possible that he had himself admitted during this time to a local mental hospital, the McLean Asylum for the Insane.[26] By August 1872,

---

[21] Diary entry, 1 February 1870, in Perry 1935a p. 322.

[22] In Feinstein p. 307.

[23] Diary entry, 30 April 1870, in James 1920a pp. 147–8.

[24] To Henry James, May 1870, in James 1920a p. 158.

[25] Feinstein p. 249.

[26] L. Menand (1998) William James and the case of the epileptic patient, *New York Review of Books* (17 December) pp. 81–3, 86–93.

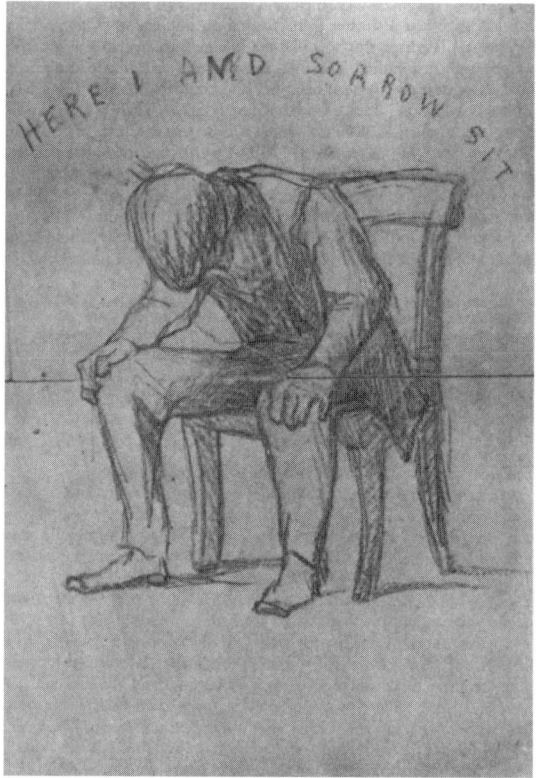

Fig. 1.4 Here I … Sorrow
Sit – by William James.

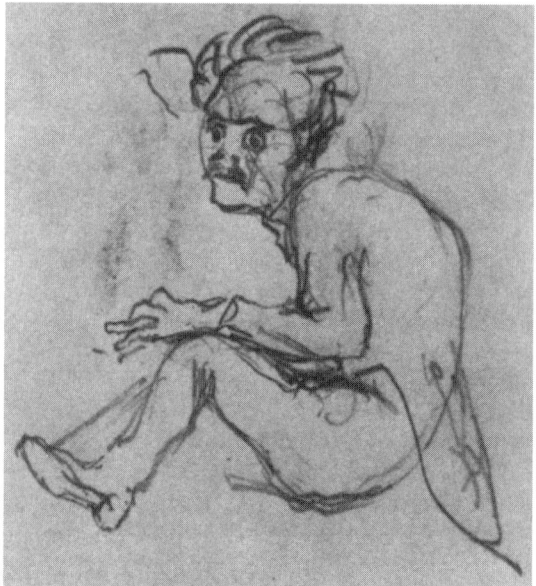

Fig. 1.5 Sitting Man – by
William James.

however, he was evidently well enough to be offered, through the help of a friend, Henry Bowditch, a teaching post in physiology at Harvard. William welcomed the job. It took his mind off what he referred to as "those introspective studies which had bred a sort of philosophical hypochondria in me of late".[27] He continued to affirm the doctrine of free will, specifically against the deterministic philosophy of Spencer, Mill, and Bain.[28] But he also continued to suffer psychologically. At about this time, he also suffered an acute episode of what he later called "panic fear",[29] which he arguably depicted in a drawing which he now did (see Fig. 1.5).[30] The next spring, he felt better. According to his father, he attributed this to learning that mental disorder is not necessarily physically determined, that the mind is free of any such deterministic coercion.[31] Nevertheless he eschewed such philosophical speculation for the certainties of science, and welcomed now being appointed to a permanent post in anatomy and physiology so much, he said, did he crave "some stable reality to lean upon".[32]

But the strain of teaching tired him, and in the autumn of 1873, he again went away, this time to Florence and Rome with his brother, Henry, who at about this time wrote a story about a man who, like William, was also chronically undecided. The story is about a man called Benvolio who is driven to distraction by self-division between love of a sociable and wealthy countess and love of the retiring daughter of a penniless professor. "It was", said Henry of Benvolio, "as if the souls of two very different men had been placed together to make the voyage of life in the same boat, and had agreed for convenience' sake to take the helm in alternation".[33] Henry's story was published in 1875. Soon after William too became divided in love.

Love, breakdown, and religion

Early in 1876 William's father came back from the Radical Club, to which both he and William belonged, announcing he had just met the woman William

---

27 To Henry James from Scarboro, 24 August 1872, in James 1920a p. 167.

28 To Charles Renouvier, from Cambridge, 2 November 1872, in James 1920a pp. 163–4.

29 W. James (1902) *The Varieties of Religious Experience*, London: Fontana, 1960 p. 166.

30 Feinstein p. 247. Feinstein argues that this episode occurred in November or early December 1872; see Feinstein p. 241.

31 From Henry James Sr to Henry James Jr, 18 March 1873, in Perry 1935a p. 340.

32 Diary entry, undated, in James 1920a p. 171.

33 H. James (1875) *Benvolio*, in L. Edel (ed.) *The Complete Tales of Henry James*, Vol. 3, London: Rupert Hart-Davis, 1962, pp. 351–401, 353.

would marry. She was a 26-year-old teacher, Alice Gibbens. Arranging through a friend, Thomas Davidson, to meet her, William soon became enthused with Alice's religious faith, and with her belief in goodness and God. Some years later he wrote approving of a friend describing her "eyes *like a prayer*". William explained "That is just the expression I have been seeking all my life".[34] Initially, however, he was plagued by uncertainty. Could he love her? Could she love him? As usual, when faced with indecision and misery, he went away. He also indicated to Alice his self-loathing. "I will suppose you feel a sympathy with me, but I can furnish you with undreamed of arguments *against* accepting any offer I may make".[35] He told her he was "split . . . into two beings", public and private, that he wished she would decide for him.[36] He wrote hoping he would learn through her "that certain goods are *real*, and compel me to live so as to merit them".[37] He told her she was his "only friend"; one who "will always stand by me and advise me and be my soul and my conscience"; that she was his "good" or "guardian angel"; that she inspired in him "things that without you would have slumbered for ever"; that she "blest" him.[38] But he was also beset by not knowing and by depression. It drained him. In early December, the same year as his involvement with Alice began, he wrote that he was living on "a little spoonful" of energy that usually gave out by mid-morning.[39]

By next April, however, he felt more confident. "Some day, God willing", he told Alice, "You shall read the bottom of my heart".[40] He felt she already "recognized" him. She made him feel that "the horrible lonesome pang is removed from my existence".[41] He admitted that he wanted to trust in his longings being fulfilled. But he also dreaded certainty making his "consciousness stagnant and stingless", unlike the "deep enthusiastic bliss" of uncertainty.[42] Perhaps all this made Alice impatient. She went away – to Canada. It left William feeling fearful that their courtship was over. But she returned.

---

[34] To Alice James, 13 May 1888, in Simon p. 155.

[35] To Alice Gibbens, September 1876, in Simon p. 159.

[36] To Alice Gibbens, 6 October 1876, in Simon p. 160.

[37] To Alice Gibbens, 9 October 1876, in Simon p.160.

[38] To Alice Gibbens, in B. Bradley (1999) From reflexivity to the need for a theory of the psychologist's life, International Society for Theoretical Psychology, Annual Conference, Sydney, Australia, 27 April.

[39] To Tom Ward, 30 December 1876, in Simon p. xiii.

[40] To Alice Gibbens, 15 April 1877, ibid. p. 160.

[41] To Alice Gibbens, 30 April 1877, ibid. p. 160.

[42] To Alice Gibbens, 7 June 1877, ibid. p. 160.

With their resumed courtship he again found himself in a "frenzy".[43] By May 1878, however, they were engaged. "Nature is too strong for all of us so I succumbed long ago", he explained to a friend, adding "Why *she* succumbed Heaven only knows but she did",[44] and on 10 July 1878 they married.

Security in love might be "stagnant and stingless", but for William the security of marriage was followed by immense productivity. He and Alice had five children.[45] The year they married saw the publication of his first signed article. In it he criticized Herbert Spencer's evolutionary determinism and doctrine of the survival of the fittest. For, said William, Spencer thereby neglected what makes survival worthwhile: love, play, art, philosophy, and, he said, "the rest of religious emotion, the joy of moral self-approbation, the charm of fancy and of wit".[46]

Now he dared increasingly to become a philosopher. In 1880 he transferred to a philosophy post in Harvard. This was followed, four years later, by the publication of his first book, arguably inspired both by love of Alice and also by love of his father. Its publication was preceded by the death, in early 1882, of William's mother, followed by the birth of William's second son, and by William suffering a nervous collapse which led to his going away to England. It was here that he learnt from his sister that their father was dying. Having been ordered by his father, *via* his sister, not to interrupt his work by coming home, William instead wrote to him:

> All my intellectual life I derive from you; and though we have often seemed at odds in the expression thereof, I'm sure there's a harmony somewhere, and that our strivings will combine. . . . You need be in no anxiety about your literary remains. I will see them well taken care of.[47]

But William's father died, on 18 December 1882, before getting William's letter. Writing of his love of his father to Alice soon after, William dwelt on his father's religious influence on him:

> For me, the humor, the good spirits, the humanity, the faith in the divine, and the sense of his right to have a say about the deepest reasons of the universe, are what will stay by me.[48]

---

[43] Ibid. p. 161.

[44] To Frances Rollins Morse, 26 May 1878, ibid. p. 162.

[45] Their children, in order of age, were Henry (born in 1879), William (born in 1882), Hermann (born in 1884), Margaret (born in 1887), and Alexander (born in 1890).

[46] W. James (1878) Remarks on Spencer's definition of mind as correspondence, in W. James (1978) *Essays in Philosophy*, Cambridge: Harvard University Press, 1978, pp. 7–12, 13, see also Simon p. 165.

[47] To Henry James Sr from Bolton Street, London, 14 December 1882, in James 1920a p. 219–20.

[48] To Alice (Gibbens) James, December 1882, ibid. p. 221.

She replied in similar vein. Her experience of his father, she told William, convinced her of "the unutterable reality, *realness, nearness* of the spiritual world".[49] Perhaps this contributed to William urging her

> You must not leave me till I understand a little more of the value and meaning of religion in Father's sense, in the mental life and destiny of man. . . . I as his son (if for no other reason) must help it to its rights in their eyes.[50]

He wrote to his mother-in-law about his father's continuing spiritual influence on him:

> It is singular how I'm learning every day now how the thought of his comments on my experiences has hitherto formed an integral part of my daily consciousness . . .
> I interrupt myself incessantly now in the old habit of imagining what he will say when I tell him this or that thing I have seen or heard.[51]

By March 1883 William had returned to Boston and the next year his promise to his father, about looking after his "literary remains", was achieved in the publication of his first book. He devoted it to his father's religious writings. In introducing them William repeated his father's account of a breakdown he had suffered, when he was 33 and staying with the then infant William and Henry, together with their mother and her sister, near Windsor Great Park in England. William's father, Henry James Sr, described his breakdown as beginning one evening, after supper, in May 1844 (when he was 32). "[I]dly gazing at the embers in the grate, thinking of nothing", he said, he became seized, "in a lightning-flash as it were", by "insane and abject terror" arising from imagining, a "damnéd shape squatting invisible to me within the precincts of the room, and raying out from his fetid personality influences fatal to life".[52]

Henry Sr attributed his recovery from this acute breakdown and his subsequent, chronic "ghastly condition of mind" which, he said, plagued him for over two years, not to the rest from work, nor to the water-cure treatment prescribed by doctors. Rather, he said, it was "spiritual medication" that made him better. He described his breakdown itself too in spiritual terms. He described it in terms borrowed from the early eighteenth century Swedish mystic, Emanuel Swedenborg, as a regenerational "vastation". Introduced by

---

[49] To William James, 1 January 1883, in Simon p. 191.

[50] To Alice (Gibbens) James, 6 January 1883, in M.E. Marty (1982) Introduction, in W. James (1902) *The Varieties of Religious Experience*, Harmondsworth: Penguin, pp. vii–xxvii, xiii.

[51] To Mrs Gibbens, February 1883, in James 1920a p. 222.

[52] In W. James (1884) Introduction, *The Literary Remains of the Late Henry James*, Boston: Houghton Mifflin, pp. 30–31.

a writer, Garth Wilkinson, who became his mentor and friend, to Swedenborg's teaching, William's father attributed his return to health to abandoning the Calvinist Presbyterianism of his father, and its assumption of separation between oneself, God, and others. Previously, he said, his will had become "fagged out" in service to this separate, alien, and "stony-hearted" figure. He only got better, he argued, thanks to his Swedenborgian "vastation", and through subsequently surrendering himself to oneness with humanity in general and with God in particular as "wholly good".[53] William put his father's breakdown and recovery in terms of his father being

> One member of that band of saints and mystics, whose . . . experience in question has always been an acute despair, passing over into an equally acute optimism, through a passion of renunciation of the self and surrender to a higher power.[54]

William evidently valued his father's account of his religious experience as a form of therapy for his previous mental suffering. But he took issue with what he called his father's "healthy-minded" focus on what is good, thereby forgetting what is bad. For this, said William, is to overlook what makes us one with those who are criminal and insane. Or, as he also put it:

> The sanest and best of us are of one clay with lunatics and prison-inmates. And whenever we feel this . . . all our morality appears but . . . the hollowest substitute for that well-*being* that our lives ought to be grounded in, but alas! Are not.[55]

As well as thus insisting on the continuity between sanity and madness, William also insisted on the continuity of consciousness. To emphasize the point he coined the term "stream of consciousness".[56] He also continued to argue in favour of asserting the will as answer to mental ill-health. In another article he announced what is now known as the James–Lange theory of the emotions. He argued that our emotions are not so much the cause as the effect of our behaviour. Changing our feelings – depression, for instance – therefore depends on exerting our will to change our behaviour:

> If we wish to conquer undesirable emotional tendencies in ourselves, we must assiduously, and in the first instance cold-bloodedly, go through the *outward motions* of those contrary dispositions we prefer to cultivate. The reward of persistency will infallibly come, in the fading out of the sullenness or depression, and the advent of real cheerfulness and kindliness in their stead.[57]

---

[53] Ibid. p. 40.

[54] Ibid. p. 37.

[55] Ibid. p. 62.

[56] W. James (1884) On some omissions of introspective psychology, *Mind*, **9** pp. 1–26, 26 n. 1.

[57] W. James (1884) What is an emotion? *Mind*, **9** pp. 188–205, 198.

James was also intrigued by divisions occurring in the will in spiritualism and hysteria.

Spiritualism and hysteria

In 1869 William James had reviewed a book about spiritualism in which he urged its scientific investigation.[58] Several years later he became involved with the founders, in 1882, of the British Society for Psychical Research (SPR) and soon helped organize an American branch. Following its first meeting in Boston in December 1884, it established a rota to investigate thought-transference, mesmerism, apparitions, divining rods, and other psychical phenomena. William James' interest in such phenomena was further increased by the death of his 18-month-old son, Hermann, on 9 July 1885, from whooping cough and pneumonia. Together with another academic, G. H. Palmer, he now started attending spiritualist seances every week, and the next year, 1886, he investigated for the SPR the trance-states of a medium called Leonora Piper.[59]

He also underwent "mind-cure" treatment involving talk, relaxation, and hypnosis. Describing it to his sister, he wrote:

> I have been paying ten or eleven visits to a mind-cure doctress, a sterling creature, resembling the "Venus of Medicine", Mrs. Lydia E. Pinkham, made solid and veracious-looking. I sit down beside her and presently drop asleep, whilst she disentangles the snarls out of my mind. She says she never saw a mind with so many, so agitated, so restless, etc. She said my *eyes*, mentally speaking, kept revolving like wheels in front of each other and in front of my face, and it was four or five sittings ere she could get them *fixed*. I am now, *unconsciously to myself*, much better than when I first went, etc. I thought it might please you to hear an opinion of my mind so similar to your own. Meanwhile what boots it to be made unconsciously better, yet all the while consciously to lie awake o'nights, as I still do?[60]

Unconfident of mind-cure therapy relieving his insomnia, he was more confident of willpower getting one up and going:

> Probably most of us have lain on certain mornings for an hour at a time unable to brace ourselves to the resolve . . . the warm couch feels too delicious, the cold outside too cruel . . . If I may generalize from my own experience, we . . . suddenly find that we *have* got up. A fortunate lapse of consciousness occurs; we forget both the warmth and the cold; we fall into some revery connected with the day's life, in the course of

[58] W. James (1869) Review of "Planchette", in G. Murphy and R. Ballou (eds) *William James on Psychical Research*, London: Chatto & Windus, 1961, pp. 19–23.

[59] W. James (1886) Report of the Committee on Mediumistic Phenomena, *Proceedings of the American Society for Psychical Research*, 1, pp. 102ff, in Murphy & Ballou pp. 95–100.

[60] To Alice James from Cambridge, 5 February 1887, in James 1920a p. 261.

which the idea flashes across us, "Hollo! I must lie here no longer" – an idea which at that lucky instant awakens no contradictory or paralyzing suggestions, and consequently produces immediately its appropriate motor effects. It was our acute consciousness of both the warmth and the cold during the period of struggle, which paralyzed our activity then and kept our idea of rising in the condition of *wish* and not of *will*. The moment these inhibitory ideas ceased, the original idea exerted its effects.[61]

By the following May, however, he felt so "fagged" out he again decided to go to Europe where he conducted thought-transference experiments with Frederic Myers and Henry Sidgwick in Cambridge, and in August met and became friends with another leading psychical researcher, Theodore Flournoy.

The same year, 1889, a book by the philosopher Pierre Janet was published, describing hysteria and the divided or weakness of the will seemingly involved in this condition. James now detailed Janet's findings. He also described Janet's account of treating hysteria through exerting his will over his patients in both hypnotizing them and getting them, under hypnosis, to recall the incidents underlying their symptoms in a happier, less traumatic light. For others "the hidden self",[62] as James called the divided-off will involved in hysteria, can, he said, be a source of transcendence and health.

James reiterated the point in his next book, *The Principles of Psychology*. In it he discussed the findings of Janet and others as evidence that, beyond what James called "primary" consciousness there lies a "secondary" consciousness. He described this secondary consciousness as a source not only of pathological "incursions" into the conscious will but also as the source of healthful incursions. "In a spiritualistic community we get optimistic messages", he wrote, adding from a Protestant viewpoint, "whilst in an ignorant Catholic village the secondary personage calls itself by the name of a demon, and proffers blasphemies and obscenities, instead of telling us how happy it is in the summer-land."[63] Together with many other issues, James also recounted further examples in his book of the will being taken over by "something more", as he put it, beyond ordinary consciousness.

He linked this further reach of the mind with immortality. In a letter to his sister, diagnosed in May 1891 with breast cancer, he wrote:

What a queer contradiction comes to the ordinary scientific argument against immortality (based on body being mind's condition and mind going *out* when body is gone),

---

61 W. James (1888) What the will effects, in W. James (1983) *Essays in Psychology*, Cambridge: Harvard University Press, 1983, pp. 216–34.

62 W. James (1890) The hidden self, *Scribner's Magazine*, 7 pp. 361–73.

63 W. James (1890) *The Principles of Psychology*, Boston: Dover, 1950, p. 228.

when one must believe (as now, in these neurotic cases) that some infernality in the body *prevents* really existing parts of the mind from coming to their effective rights at all, suppresses them, and blots them out from participation in this world's experiences, although they are *there* all the time.[64]

He also taught a seminar on abnormal psychology, emphasizing, as he had before, "that there is no sharp line to be drawn between 'healthy' and 'unhealthy' minds, that all have something of both".[65]

Religious therapy

William James now began focusing on the mental health benefits of religious belief. In a lecture to the Yale Philosophy Club on 17 April 1896 he argued that whenever we are unable to choose, on intellectual grounds, between different courses of action we should be guided by our will. This also applies, he said, in choosing whether or not to believe in God. Given the benefits of such belief, he argued, it is better to believe than not.[66]

Whether or not James succeeded in willing himself to believe, he was cut off from religious experience. He also found himself cut off from the mystical experience others often find through taking mescalin. Whereas a therapist colleague, Weir Mitchell, promised it would give him "glorious visions of colour", he complained it simply made him "violently sick".[67] He was nevertheless convinced that mystical and religious experience could cure depression and self-division:

> After the conversion crisis, the higher loves and powers come definitively to gain the upper-hand and expel the forces which up to that time had kept them down in the position of mere grumblers and protesters and agents of remorse and discontent.[68]

He also defended religious therapy against those in the Massachusetts legislature wanting to outlaw people without medical degrees practising as psychotherapists. Of mind-cure and Christian Science therapy, he reported,

> They are proving by the most brilliant new results that the therapeutic relation may be what we can at present describe only as a relation of one person to another . . . Their movement is a religious or quasi-religious movement . . . [in which] impressions and intuitions seem to accomplish more than chemical, anatomical or physiological information.[69]

---

[64] To his sister, Alice, 6 July 1891, in James 1920a pp. 310–1 – emphasis in original.

[65] H. James (1920b) *The Letters of William James, Vol. II*, Boston: Atlantic Monthly Press, p. 15.

[66] W. James (1896) The will to believe, in W. James (1897) *The Will to Believe*, New York: Dover, 1956, pp. 1–31.

[67] To Henry James from Chocorua, 11 June 1896, in James 1920b p. 37.

[68] To Henry Rankin from Newport, Rhode Island, 1 February 1897, ibid. p. 57.

[69] March 1898, ibid. pp. 69, 71.

Later that summer, 1898, he himself had a quasi-religious conversion experience after falling in love, it seems, with a young woman, Pauline Goldmark,
whilst on holiday in the Adirondacks.

> The influences of Nature, the wholesomeness of the people round me, especially the
> good Pauline . . . fermented within me till it became a regular Walpurgis Nacht. I spent
> a good deal of it in the woods, where the streaming moonlight lit up things in a magi-
> cal checkered play, and it seemed as if the Gods of all the nature-mythologies were
> holding an indescribable meeting in my breast with the moral Gods of the inner life.[70]

Such revelations, he said, are the inspiration of organized religion: "What
keeps religion going", he maintained in a lecture in Berkeley that August, is not
academic theology but "religious experiences . . . in the lives of humble private
men . . . conversations with the unseen, voices and visions, responses to
prayer, changes of heart, deliverances from fear, inflowings of help, assurances
of support".[71]

The next summer he became ill with irreparable damage to his heart following a "thirteen-hours' scramble" after losing his way walking and climbing in
the mountains near his New Hampshire home, Chocorua. He went for treatment to Europe. Here he worked on the Gifford Lectures which he had been
invited to give in Scotland, but which had been postponed because of his
heart-trouble. He told a friend that, in the lectures, he would not dwell on
theology and religious doctrine but on the immediacy of religious experience
as, what he called, "the real backbone of the world's religious life".[72] But he was
also still enthusiastic about the will, as means of conquering depression.[73]

In his lectures, however, he planned not so much to emphasize exerting the
will as surrendering it to "irruptions" from the "extended subliminal self".[74]
The lectures began on 16 May 1901, and were published the next June as
a book, *The Varieties of Religious Experience*. It begins with James's pragmatism and individualism. He warned his readers that he judged religious experience by its "fruits",[75] and that he was not concerned with collective or organized
religion but with "the feelings, acts, and experiences of individual men in their
solitude, so far as they apprehend themselves to stand in relation to whatever

----

[70] To Alice (Gibbens) James from St. Hubert's Inn, Keene Valley, 9 July 1898, ibid. p. 76.

[71] In R. B. Perry (1935b) *The Thought and Character of William James, Vol. II*, p. 325.

[72] To Miss Frances Morse from Costebelle, 12 April 1900, in James 1920b p. 127.

[73] Letter to his daughter, Margaret, from Villa Luise, Bad-Nauheim, 26 May 1900, ibid.
      p. 131–2.

[74] To Henry Rankin from Edinburgh, 16 June 1901, ibid. p. 149.

[75] James 1902 p. 41.

they consider divine".[76] To this he added that by "divine" he meant non-theistic as well as theistic, Buddhist as well as Christian religious experience, whatever "is god*like*", he said, "whether it be a concrete deity or not".[77] The essence of the religious life, he maintained, entails adjusting to an unseen order believed to constitute our "supreme good".[78]

He evoked the inspiring sense of the presence of, and oneness with this goodness – or God – with examples collected by himself and other researchers. He quoted, for instance, a clergyman writing

> I remember the night, and almost the very spot on the hill-top, where my soul opened out, as it were, into the Infinite, and there was a rushing together of the two worlds, the inner and the outer . . . I stood alone with Him who had made me, and all the beauty of the world, and love, and sorrow, and even temptation. I did not seek Him, but felt the perfect unison of my spirit with His.[79]

Another example came from James' psychical researcher friend and colleague, Theodore Flournoy: "All at once I experience a feeling of being raised above myself, I felt the presence of God . . . as if his goodness and power were penetrating me altogether".[80]

James likened these experiences to those of the oneness with, and presence of one's beloved: "A lover has notoriously this sense of the continuous being of his idol . . . He cannot forget her; she uninterruptedly affects him through and through."[81] He also quoted from an 1899 book about mind-cure philosophy:

> The great central fact in human life is the coming into a conscious vital realization of our oneness with this Infinite Life, and the opening of ourselves fully to this divine inflow . . . In just the degree in which you realize your oneness with the Infinite Spirit, you will exchange dis-ease for ease, inharmony for harmony, suffering and pain for abounding health and strength.[82]

Generalizing from this and other examples, James said mind-cure and Christian Science therapists were governed by belief in the all-saving power of "healthy-minded" attitudes – "courage, hope, and trust" – and by contempt for their antithesis – "doubt, fear, worry, and all nervously precautionary states of mind".[83]

[76] James 1902 p. 31.

[77] Ibid. p. 53, see also D. Scott (2000) William James and Buddhism, *Religion*, **30** pp. 333–52.

[78] Ibid. 1902 p. 69.

[79] Ibid. p. 81.

[80] Ibid. p. 82.

[81] Ibid. p. 87.

[82] Ibid. pp. 112, 113.

[83] Ibid. p. 107.

According to this philosophy, he wrote, "we are already one with the Divine without any miracle of grace, or abrupt creation of a new inner man".[84] As an example of someone successfully treated by this approach, James quoted a woman describing herself as follows before and after therapy:

> Life seemed difficult to me at one time. I was always breaking down, and had several attacks of what is called nervous prostration . . . I never recovered permanently till this New Thought took possession of me. . . . the fact that we must be in absolutely constant relation or mental touch (this word is to me very expressive) with that essence of life which permeates all and which we call God . . . by a constant turning to the very innermost, deepest consciousness of our real selves or of God in us, for illumination from within, just as we turn to the sun for light, warmth, and invigoration without.[85]

From the optimism of mind-cure therapy, James turned to the pessimism of what he called "the sick soul" – of those who, he said, feel that "good has no reality".[86] As illustration he described a hospitalized, suicidal patient "so choked with the feeling of evil", said James, "that the sense of there being any good in the world is lost for him altogether".[87] James also recounted his own experience, from his late 20s or early 30s, of panic fear:

> Whilst in this state of philosophic pessimism and general depression of spirits about my prospects, I went one evening into a dressing-room in the twilight to procure some article that was there; when suddenly there fell upon me without any warning, just as if it came out of the darkness, a horrible fear of my own existence. Simultaneously there arose in my mind the image of an epileptic patient whom I had seen in the asylum, a black-haired youth with greenish skin, entirely idiotic, who used to sit all day on one of the benches, or rather shelves against the wall, with his knees drawn up against his chin and the coarse gray undershirt, which was his only garment, drawn over them, inclosing his entire figure. He sat there like a sort of sculptured Egyptian cat or Peruvian mummy, moving nothing but his black eyes and looking absolutely non-human. This image and my fear entered into a species of combination with each other. *That shape am I*, I felt, potentially. Nothing that I possess can defend me against that fate, if the hour for it should strike for me as it struck for him. There was such a horror of him, and such a perception of my own merely momentary discrepancy from him, that it was as if something hitherto solid within my breast gave way entirely, and I became a mass of quivering fear. After this the universe was changed for me altogether. I awoke morning after morning with a horrible dread at the pit of my stomach, and with a sense of the insecurity of life that I never knew before, and that I have never felt since. It was like a revelation; and although the immediate feelings

----

84 Ibid. p. 112.

85 Ibid. p. 114.

86 Ibid. p. 152.

87 Ibid. p. 156.

passed away, the experience has made me sympathetic with the morbid feelings of others ever since. It gradually faded, but for months I was unable to go out into the dark alone.[88]

He related this incident to the similar terrifying episode experienced by his father in Windsor in his early 30s (see p. 18 above).[89]

William James described such experiences as constituted by alienating self-division between good and bad, or, more generally, between our ideal and actual self. Religious experience, he said, is particularly valuable in treating such division. Through sudden or gradual religious conversion, transformation, grace, or regeneration, he said, "a self hitherto divided, and consciously wrong, inferior and unhappy, becomes unified and consciously right, superior and happy, in consequence of its firmer hold upon religious realities".[90] As illustration he quoted a man, Stephen Bradley, saying of his religious conversion experience, occurring in November 1829:

> I began to be exercised by the Holy Spirit . . . My heart seemed as if it would burst, but it did not stop until I felt as if I was unutterably full of the love and grace of God.[91]

Such conversions or transformations, said James, are due to influences working "subconsciously or half unconsciously".[92] They entail surrendering the will to these influences. He illustrated the point with another example, Henry Alline, who, describing his religious transformation, occurring in March 1775, wrote:

> At that instant of time when I gave all up to him to do with me as he pleased, and was willing that God should rule over me at his pleasure, redeeming love broke into my soul with repeated scriptures, with such power that my whole soul seemed to be melted down with love . . . my whole soul, that was a few minutes ago groaning under mountains of death, and crying to an unknown God for help, was now filled with immortal love.[93]

Nevertheless, said James, Alline, like others, was one of those "upon whose soul the iron of melancholy left a permanent imprint" even after their religious conversion experience.[94] He called them the "twice-born".

....

[88] James 1902 pp. 166–7. Although James recounted the experience as though it was that of someone else – a Frenchman – when he was asked about it, in 1904, by its translator into French, Frank Abauzit, a friend of Theodore Flournoy, James admitted it was his "own case" – in Menand p. 81.

[89] James 1902 p. 168 n. 1.

[90] Ibid. p. 194.

[91] Ibid. p. 196.

[92] Ibid. p. 202.

[93] Ibid. p. 220.

[94] Ibid. p. 222.

Generalizing, he detailed the positive and therapeutic effects of religious experience: the sense of higher control; immediate and intuitive sense of salvation, faith, and trust; freedom from worry; peace in simply being; the sense of perceiving truths not previously known; appearance of newness in everything; and "photism" involving actual or metaphorical sense of illumination and light. James also wrote of the "ecstasy of happiness" of religious conversion experience.[95] He likened it to being in love, maintaining that in both cases the intensity diminishes, but not necessarily their revelations.

Under the heading of "saintliness", James outlined both excesses and benefits of religious experience, including "equanimity, receptivity, and peace" through casting off the "burden" of willing and doing.[96] He also described the following characteristics of mystical experience: "ineffable" in being beyond words; "noetic" in bringing about insight "unplumbed by the discursive intellect";[97] transience; and passivity with the mystic feeling "as if he were grasped and held by a superior power".[98]

James also described means of achieving mystical experience through detaching one's mind from "outer sensations",[99] and through emptying oneself as noted by St Paul, saying "Only when I become as nothing can God enter in",[100] and as noted in another book about mysticism:

> The treasure of treasures for the soul is where she goeth out of the Somewhat into that Nothing out of which all things may be made. The soul here saith, *I have nothing . . . I can do nothing . . . I am nothing . . .* so God may will all in me.[101]

Through thus achieving mystical states of mind, wrote James, "we both become one with the Absolute and we become aware of our oneness".[102] Achievement of this experience, he went on, depends on having "an active subliminal self" and on our openness to being ready to receive the "higher spiritual agencies" it transmits, just as our "primary wide-awake consciousness" opens our senses to material reality.[103] He added:

> If the word "subliminal" is offensive to any of you, as smelling too much of psychical research, call it by any other name you please, to distinguish it from the level of full

95 Ibid. p. 253.

96 Ibid. p. 285.

97 Ibid. p. 367.

98 Ibid. p. 368.

99 Ibid. p. 392.

100 Ibid. p. 403.

101 Ibid. p. 403.

102 Ibid. p. 404.

103 Ibid. p. 242.

sunlit consciousness. Call this latter the A-region of personality, if you care to, and call the other the B-region.[104]

He described the B-region as "the abode of everything that is latent". It is, he said, the source of our "intuitions . . . all our non-rational operations . . . [and] dreams".[105] It is unconscious. It is not aware of itself. Rather, he said, it provides material for the concepts of reflecting and thinking. It constitutes, he told Henri Bergson, the "subconscious" equivalent of the "soul".[106]

Having dwelt on the mental health benefits of religious and mystical experience, James regretted having little personal experience of it. "I have no living commerce with God", he wrote, adding "I envy those who have, for I know the addition of such a sense would help me immensely".[107] But he feared lest, were he to suspend his will and open himself to his unconscious or subliminal self, demonic evil rather than divine good might emerge. He dreaded lest, like a case of multiple personality described by the psychiatrist, Morton Prince, he too might become subject to a will alien and hostile to his own. Worried that he had indeed become invaded by the dreams of someone else one night in February 1906, he feared that surrendering his will would result in his being "swept out to sea with no horizon and no bond".[108]

Nevertheless he remained sympathetic to mysticism and to what he called "Yoga practices" as "methods of getting at our deeper functional levels" akin to "religious crises . . . love-crises, etc.".[109] He was also supportive of the self-help mental health movement led by Clifford Beers and others. In lectures in Oxford and elsewhere he also continued to emphasize the value of religious experience through surrendering one's will and "letting something higher work for us".[110] He was accordingly appalled by Freud reportedly rejecting "American religious therapy" as unscientific despite what James called its "extensive results".[111] Nevertheless he also emphasized that Freud's ideas "can't fail to throw light on human nature".[112] Warmly putting his arm around Freud

---

[104] James 1902 p. 462.

[105] Ibid. p. 462.

[106] To Henri Bergson from Cambridge, 25 February 1903, in James 1920b p. 184.

[107] To James Leuba from Cambridge, 17 April 1904, ibid. p. 211.

[108] W. James (1910) A suggestion about mysticism, in *Philosophy*, Cambridge: Harvard University Press, 1978, pp. 157–66, 162.

[109] To W. Lutoslawski from Cambridge, 6 May 1906, in James 1920b p. 254.

[110] W. James (1909) *A Pluralistic Universe*, New York: Longmans, Green & Co., p. 305.

[111] To Theodore Flournoy from Chocorua, 28 September 1909, in James 1920b pp. 327–8.

[112] Ibid. p. 328.

when he visited Massachusetts in 1909, James told him "the future of psychology belongs to your work".[113] Freud was likewise warm in his subsequent memories of James:

> I shall never forget one little scene that occurred as we were on a walk together. He stopped suddenly, handed me a bag he was carrying and asked me to walk on, saying that he would catch me up as soon as he had gone through an attack of angina pectoris which was just coming on. He died of that disease a year later; and I have always wished that I might be as fearless as he was in the face of approaching death.[114]

Whatever Freud's reservations about religious and what would now be called "alternative" therapy, James remained an enthusiast till the end. He had treatment from a Christian Scientist, L. G. Strang, in late 1904,[115] and in his final months had homeopathic treatment for anxiety and insomnia. He also continued doing psychical research, attended a spiritualist seance in Paris, and went to see his psychical researcher friend and colleague, Flournoy, in Geneva during his last visit to Europe in 1910. In July he returned with his brother, Henry, and his wife, Alice, to their New Hampshire home where he died the next month, on 26 August 1910.

After William's death Alice held spiritualist seances in their home. Meanwhile Henry returned to England and to his writing career, of which he wrote to a fellow-novelist:

> We must know, as much as possible, in our beautiful art, yours & mine, what we are talking about – & the only way to know it is to have lived & loved & cursed and floundered & enjoyed & suffered – I think I don't regret a single "excess" of my responsive youth – I only regret, in my chilled age, certain occasions & possibilities I didn't embrace.[116]

William, too, embraced experience, including experimenting with laughing gas and other means to secure religious and mystical experience. Freud too embraced experience. But it led to a quite different conclusion, to the founding of a therapy – psychoanalysis – that was initially entirely hostile to religion.

---

[113] In E. Jones (1958) *Sigmund Freud, Vol. II*, London: Hogarth, p. 64.

[114] In K. Townsend (1996) *Manhood at Harvard*, New York: Norton, p. 285.

[115] Simon p. 376.

[116] To Hugh Walpole, in P. Horne (2002) Review of *Dearly Beloved Friends: Henry James's Letters to Younger Men*, Minneapolis: University of Michigan Press, *Times Literary Supplement*, 24 May, p. 13.

Chapter 2

Sigmund Freud

Freeing love

Whereas William James argued that religious experience, mediated by the unconscious, helps people become whole and well, Sigmund Freud rejected religion and religious experience because he believed that they contributed to women and men remaining or becoming unconscious of the truth, including the truth of sex and love. Later, in part because of disappointments in love, Freud betrayed the truth of both love and mystical experience in rejecting the oneness involved in them as an illusion. I will explain all this later in this chapter, after detailing the loves accompanying and inspiring his insights in founding psychoanalysis – in which he said scarcely anything about religion. I will preface this, however, by first recounting his earlier involvement with both it and religion.

Early science and religion

Freud was born in Freiberg on 6 May 1856. By then his father, Jacob, an impecunious wool-merchant already had two grown-up sons (Emmanuel and Philipp) by his first marriage. Freud's birth was followed by the birth of seven more children.[1] Meanwhile, because of growing anti-semitism in Catholic Freiberg during the 1859 Austro-Italian war, Jacob took the family that year to Leipzig, and the next year to Vienna, where they settled in a Jewish area, Leopoldstadt.

Freud later attributed his pursuit of truth whatever its consequences to his minority status as a Jew in predominantly Catholic Vienna. It freed him, he said, from many "prejudices which restricted others in the use of their intellect", thereby early preparing him "to join the opposition" and do without "agreement with the 'compact majority'".[2] He was brought up in the Jewish faith. Although his father eventually dispensed with all religious observances – except Purim and Passover – he continued to read the Talmud and Torah in the holy language – Hebrew – and this inspired Freud to become engrossed in

---

[1] Julius, who died soon after he was born, Anna, who was born when Freud was 2, Rosa, Marie, Adolphine, Pauline, and Alexander, born when Freud was 10 and named, at his suggestion, after Alexander the Great.

[2] S. Freud (1914) On the history of the psychoanalytic movement, **SE14** pp. 3–66, 14.

"the Bible story", as he later put it, "almost as soon as I had learnt the art of reading".[3] Many years later his father recalled Freud's childhood in religious terms, in inscribing in a Bible he gave him:

> It was in the seventh year of your age that the spirit of God began to move you to learning. I would say the spirit of God speaketh to you: "Read in My Book; there will be opened to thee sources of knowledge and of the intellect". It is the Book of Books.[4]

When he went to secondary school Freud was also taught Hebrew and the Jewish religion by Samuel Hammerschlag, who became a close friend.

Here he was inspired by science, particularly, as he put it, by "hearing Goethe's beautiful essay on Nature read aloud at a popular lecture by Professor Carl Brühl".[5] It decided him to study medicine because, he said, he was more interested in people than in things. Or, as he also put it, he "felt an overwhelming need to understand something of the riddles of the world in which we live and perhaps even to contribute something to their solution".[6] He accordingly registered, on leaving school in 1873, to study medicine at the University of Vienna. Here – as well as taking courses in anatomy, chemistry, and physiology – he also took classes in philosophy with an ex-priest, Franz Brentano, of which he wrote "I, the godless medical man and empiricist, am attending two courses in philosophy and reading Feuerbach in Paneth's company. One of the courses – listen and marvel! – deals with the existence of God".[7]

Freud particularly admired Feuerbach, and perhaps it was from Feuerbach's argument that reason exposes religion to be an illusion that Freud learnt to later dismiss religion in similar terms. "For the time being", however, he wrote of Brentano's religious teaching, "I have ceased to be a materialist and am not yet a theist".[8] But he was fearful:

> Ever since Brentano adduced such ridiculously simple arguments in favor of his God, I have been afraid that one fine day I will be taken in by the scientific proofs of the validity of spiritualism, homeopathy, by Louise Lateau [a young woman who had apparently manifested the stigmata], etc.[9]

He was particularly disturbed, he said, by Brentano's arguments persuading him that the "science of all things seems to demand the existence of God".[10]

---

[3] S. Freud (1925) An autobiographical study, **SE20** pp. 7–74, 8.

[4] In E. Jones (1961) *The Life and Work of Sigmund Freud*, London: Penguin, p. 47.

[5] Freud 1925 p. 8.

[6] In Jones 1961 p. 54.

[7] To Silberstein, 8 November 1874, in W. Boehlich (1990) *The Letters of Sigmund Freud to Eduard Silberstein 1871–1881*, Cambridge: Harvard University Press, p. 70.

[8] To Silberstein, 15 March 1875, ibid. pp. 104–5.

[9] To Silberstein, 27 March 1875, ibid. p. 106.

[10] To Silberstein, 11 April 1875, ibid. p. 111.

Most of all his commitment was to science and to research. Soon after doing comparative anatomy research in Trieste in 1876 he joined Ernst Brücke's physiology research institute in Vienna. It was here that he first met Josef Breuer.

Inspiring loves

Josef Breuer was slightly older than Freud and became one of the first loves inspiring his earliest discoveries in psychoanalysis. Later he wrote of Breuer that being with him was

> Like sitting in the sun . . . he radiates light and warmth . . . One does not adequately characterize him by saying only good things about him; one has also to emphasize the absence of so much badness.[11]

Like Breuer, Freud too became a doctor (in March 1881), continued his physiology research, and in the spring of 1882, fell in love with the sister of one of his school-friends, Eli Bernays.

Martha Bernays was 22 when Freud first noticed her visiting his family on his return from work one day in April 1882. Instead of going to his room to study as he usually did, he stayed on with her and the family. Like his family, Martha too was Jewish. But, unlike his family, hers were strictly orthodox Jews. As Chief Rabbi of Hamburg, Martha's grandfather, Isaac Bernays, had opposed the Jewish reform movement there. Her father had brought the family to Vienna in 1869 to work for an economist there but had suddenly died from heart failure in early December 1879.

Now, nearly three years later, on 17 June 1882, Martha and Freud became secretly engaged. The next day Martha returned with her mother to the family's home town, Wandsbek, near Hamburg. This was immediately followed by Freud writing the first of more than nine hundred letters to her during their over four years' long engagement:

> My precious, most beloved girl . . . I still cannot grasp it, and if that elegant little box and that sweet picture were not lying in front of me, I would think it was all a beguiling dream and be afraid to wake up. Yet friends tell me it's true, and I myself can remember details more charming, more mysteriously enchanting than any dream-phantasy could create. It must be true. Martha is mine, the sweet girl of whom everyone speaks with admiration, who despite all my resistance captivated my heart at our first meeting . . . When you return, darling girl . . . we will talk of the time when there will be no difference between night and day, when neither intrusions from without nor farewells nor worries shall keep us apart.[12]

---

[11] In Jones 1961 pp. 160, 161, see also W. Koestenbaum (1989) *Double Talk: The Erotics of Male Literary Collaboration*, London: Routledge.

[12] To Martha Bernays, 19 June 1882, in E. Freud (1961) *Letters of Sigmund Freud 1873–1939*, London: Hogarth, pp. 25, 26.

Longing to marry Martha, and advised by Brücke that, since he had no other means of support, he should get better paid work, Freud reluctantly gave up doing research and, after visiting Martha for a couple of days in July 1882, started work the next month in internal medicine in Vienna's general hospital where, the next May, he transferred to work in psychiatry. Martha returned to Vienna in September 1882, but again went back to Wandsbek the next summer. Freud's letters to her there included one about Breuer's treatment of a friend of hers, Berthe Pappenheim, now known in psychoanalytic history as Anna O, and as inventor, with Breuer, of "the talking cure". This included her telling Breuer her half-waking nightmares and dreams, just as Freud told Martha his:

> My beloved Marty . . . Continually having so much to do acts as a kind of narcotic, but as you know I have lately been looking for something to rescue me from my great emotional and excitable state. . . . Strange creatures are billeted in my brain. . . . [But when] a letter from you arrives the whole dream fades, life enters my cell. Then all the strange problems creep away, the mysterious pictures of diseases fade, and gone are the empty theories "according to the present status of science", as they are invariably called. Then the world turns so warm, so gay, so easy to understand. My sweet darling is no illusion, she does not have to be proved by chemical tests; in fact she can, although no giant, be seen by the naked eye. Fortunately she has nothing to do with diseases – I hope she is very well – except that she was incautious enough to take a doctor for a lover. Oh Marty, it is so much more lovely to be a human being than a warehouse for certain monotonous experiences. But one is not allowed to be a human being for an hour unless one has been a machine or a warehouse for eleven hours.[13]

The same month Martha's brother, Eli, married Freud's sister, Anna. Perhaps this contributed to Freud pining for Martha – "I have been thinking of you more than usual during these past days".[14] On seeing Raphael's *Sistine Madonna* in Dresden the next month he yearned

> Oh, if only you were with me! . . . The painting emanates a magic beauty that is inescapable . . . she gazes out on the world with such a fresh and innocent expression . . . not from the celestial world but from ours.[15]

Further love letters followed his appointment, in early 1884, to work as a neurologist. He quoted Schiller to Martha – "Hunger and love: that, after all, is the true philosophy".[16] He told her of his friendship with Ernst von Fleischl-Marxow, whom he had first got to know when he was a research physiologist,

---

[13] To Martha Bernays, 9 October 1883, in Freud 1961 pp. 82, 83.

[14] To Martha Bernays, 15 November 1883, in Freud 1961 p. 89.

[15] To Martha Bernays, 20 December 1883, in Freud 1961 pp. 96, 97.

[16] To Martha Bernays, 12 February 1884, in P. Gay (1988) *Freud*, London: Macmillan, p. 46.

"I love him not so much as a human being", Freud told her, "but as one of Creation's precious achievements".[17] He told her of his planned experiments with cocaine, a drug he recommended to Fleischl in the hope that it would relieve him of his morphine addiction.

The next spring he started working in opthalomology, taught neuropathology and, from early June 1885, also worked in a private mental hospital just outside Vienna. Wanting to learn more about the then renowned discoveries of Jean Martin Charcot in treating hysteria at the Salpêtrière hospital in Paris, he applied for a travel grant to go there. Meanwhile he still longed for Martha. "My beloved little woman", he wrote to her

> I have been yearning for you recently more than I ever have since that first time we were forced to separate. This is the result of your sweet tender letter which I carry with me wherever I go. I am so boundlessly happy about it . . . I just cannot find the right words. I would rather dwell on how fast the next $2\frac{1}{2}$ months are going to pass . . . the travelling grant, . . . is terribly important to me, although no longer quite so urgent as at the time when my coming to you depended exclusively on this decision. I dream about this grant every night; yesterday for instance I dreamt that Brücke told me I couldn't get it, that there were seven other applicants, all of whom had greater chances![18]

The next day success. He won the grant, he told Martha, 13 votes to 8, adding:

> Princess, my little princess. Oh, how wonderful it will be! I am coming with money and staying a long time . . . and then we will soon get married . . . and I will go on kissing you till you are strong and gay and happy . . . I am quite unspeakably happy. June really is a kind month.[19]

He spent almost all September with Martha on his way to Paris where, as well as studying with Charcot, he did research on children's brains. He enthused to Martha about Charcot, about his "lively interest" in everything,[20] about his being "one of the greatest of physicians" adding "I sometimes come out of his lectures as from out of Notre-Dame, with an entirely new idea about perfection".[21] After spending Christmas with Martha, he returned to Paris where he worked on translating Charcot's lectures. Particularly inspiring was the fact that, whereas others dismissed hysteria as mere effect of the imagination, Charcot took it seriously precisely on this score. He argued that hysteria is both caused psychologically – by trauma – and that it can be cured

---

[17] In Jones 1961 p. 100.

[18] To Martha Bernays, 19 June 1885, in Freud 1961 pp. 165, 166.

[19] To Martha Bernays, 20 June 1885, in Freud 1961 p. 166.

[20] To Martha Bernays, 21 October 1885, in Freud 1961 p. 187.

[21] To Martha Bernays, 24 November 1885, in Freud 1961 p. 196.

psychologically – through hypnosis. Freud also very much admired Charcot's approach to research:

> He had the nature of an artist – he was, as he himself said, a '*visuel*', a man who sees . . . He used to look again and again at the things he did not understand, to deepen his impression of them day by day, till suddenly an understanding of them dawned on him. In his mind's eye the apparent chaos presented by the continual repetition of the same symptoms then gave way to order: the new nosological pictures emerged.[22]

Freud was also impressed by Charcot's insight into the origin of mental illness in sex and love. Years later he still recalled overhearing Charcot, at a reception in his home, attributing a young woman's nervous symptoms to her husband's sexual awkwardness or impotence, emphasizing "*Mais, dans des cas pareils c'est toujours la chose génitale, toujours . . . toujours . . . toujours*".[23]

By late February 1886, however, Freud had to leave Charcot and Paris. After a brief visit to Martha, followed by three weeks' study of children's diseases in Berlin, he returned to Vienna, where he placed an advertisement in that Easter Sunday's paper announcing the start of his private practice as a doctor specializing in nervous diseases. In August he had to do a month's military service. Then, thanks to money from one of Martha's aunts, they could at last marry, which they did on 13 September 1886. The wedding had to be followed by a religious ceremony. But Freud refused, from the very first Friday of their marriage, to allow Martha to light the Sabbath lights that evening. Settled in Vienna, they soon had six children, all named after men, or after the female relatives of men Freud particularly admired.[24]

Soon after the birth of their first child, Mathilde, in October 1887, Freud began a correspondence with a fellow-doctor, Wilhelm Fliess who, more than anyone else, inspired his first development of psychoanalysis. Born in 1858, Fliess was an ear, nose, and throat specialist in Berlin, who came to study in Vienna where, on Breuer's recommendation, he went to Freud's lectures. Soon after his return to Berlin, Freud wrote to him:

> Esteemed friend and colleague: My letter of today admittedly is occasioned by business; but I must introduce it by confessing that I entertain hopes of continuing the relationship with you and that you have left a deep impression on me.[25]

---

22 S. Freud (1893) Charcot, **SE3** pp. 11–23, 12.

23 S. Freud (1914) On the history of the psycho-analytic movement, **SE14** pp. 3–66, 14.

24 Mathilde (born on 16 October 1887) was named after Breuer's wife; Martin (born on 6 October 1889) was named after Charcot; Oliver (born on 19 February 1891) was named after Cromwell; Ernst (born on 6 April 1892) was named after Brücke; Sophie (born on 12 April 1893) was named after Hammerschlag's niece; and Anna (born on 3 December 1895) was named after Hammerschlag's daughter.

25 To Fliess, 24 November 1887, in J. Masson (1985) *The Complete Letters of Sigmund Freud to Wilhelm Fliess 1887–1904*, Cambridge: Harvard University Press, p. 15.

Fliess responded by sending Freud a present. It was "magnificent", said Freud, "I still do not know how I won you . . . But I am very happy about it".[26]

He also told Fliess about the method of treatment he was using with his patients. Previously he had used electrotherapy. Now, he said, he was using hypnotism. Soon he began combining it with what he later called "free association". In May 1889 he described a patient, Emmy von N, freely associating "memories and new impressions" affecting her since they had last met, which in turn led to

> Pathogenic reminiscences of which she unburdens herself without being asked to . . . as though she had adopted my procedure and was making use of our conversation, apparently unconstrained and guided by chance, as a supplement to her hypnosis.[27]

The same year Freud went to Nancy to study hypnotism with Hippolyte Bernheim. Just as William James was impressed by Janet's findings using hypnotism with hysterical patients, so Freud was impressed with Bernheim's findings. They gave him, he said, "the profoundest impression of the possibility that there could be powerful mental processes which nevertheless remained hidden from the consciousness of man".[28]

Meanwhile his involvement with Fliess was deepening. He was delighted by Fliess's suggestion that they meet:

> Your invitation is the loveliest thing and the greatest honor that has happened to me in a long time. I very much look forward to seeing you again, to hearing what you are up to, and to rekindling my almost extinguished energy and scientific interests on yours.[29]

But a few days later Freud wrote disconsolately cancelling the meeting, saying "my wife who otherwise never wants to stand in the way of small trips really dislikes this particular one".[30] Within ten days, however, it was agreed they could meet. "Dearest friend", wrote Freud, "Splendid! And do you know of anywhere more lovely than Salzburg for this purpose? We will meet there and hike for a few days wherever you want".[31] He sent Fliess his first book (about aphasia), met with him during his visits to Vienna to see his fiancée, Ida Bondy, and soon after their marriage, began addressing Fliess as "*du*" in a letter in which he also announced Breuer's agreement to their publishing a joint

---

[26] To Fliess, 28 December 1887, ibid. p. 16.

[27] S. Freud and J. Breuer (1895) *Studies on Hysteria*, **SE2** p. 56.

[28] Freud 1925 p. 17.

[29] To Fliess, 21 July 1890, in Masson p. 26.

[30] To Fliess, 1 August 1890, ibid. p. 27.

[31] To Fliess, 11 August 1890, ibid. pp. 27–8.

account of their discoveries about treating hysteria.[32] It included Freud's account of supplementing hypnosis with the following technique:

> After asking a patient some question such as: "How long have you had this symptom?" or: "What was its origin?" . . . I placed my hands on the patient's forehead or took her head between my hands and said: "You will think of it under the pressure of my hand. At the moment at which I relax my pressure you will see something in front of you or something will come into your head. Catch hold of it. It will be what we are looking for. – Well, what have you seen or what has occurred to you?"[33]

Using this technique with one of his patients, a 30-year-old English governess whom he began treating at the end of 1892, Freud found that her symptoms – including a persistent smell of burnt pudding – were relieved by the technique revealing that they were a somatic means of representing her repressed love for her employer. Through therapy enabling her to become fully conscious of her love, she could begin to think about it emotionally in words rather than express it unthinkingly in the bodily symptoms of hysteria for which she had sought treatment from Freud.

In reporting their findings Freud and Breuer argued that hysteria is not due to trauma itself, but to the memory of trauma. Treatment of hysteria accordingly entails dissolving the resistance to recalling this memory to consciousness so that the feelings associated with the trauma can be experienced and thought about consciously, rather than remaining dissociated from ordinary consciousness. Breuer and Freud attributed this dissociation to the circumstances attending the trauma's first occurrence, to its occurring when the patient was in what Breuer called a "hypnoid" state, or to the patient repressing the trauma and its associated feelings.[34]

Freud favoured the latter explanation. He had noticed that the feelings involved often concerned the patient's love life. An example was a young woman, Elisabeth von R, whom Freud pressed to report "faithfully", as he put it, "whatever appeared before her inner eye or passed through her memory at the moment of the pressure" of his hand on her head.[35] This revealed that her symptoms – pains in her legs and difficulties in walking – expressed in bodily terms her defence against her unconscious wish that her sister die so she could marry her husband. Her treatment freed this wish from repression so it could be consciously experienced and thought about. The result, said Freud, was the

[32] To Fliess, 28 June 1892, ibid. p. 31.

[33] S. Freud (1895) in S. Freud and J. Breuer (1895) *Studies on Hysteria*, SE2, p. 110.

[34] S. Freud and J. Breuer (1893) On the psychical mechanism of hysterical phenomena, SE2 pp. 3–17, 12.

[35] In Freud and Breuer p. 145 (see n. 26 above).

first case of a complete "psychical analysis".[36] Generalizing from this success, Freud wrote an essay, a draft of which he sent to Fliess, in which he emphasized that neurosis is due to the repression of sex, and that mental health therefore entails freeing it through, for instance, developing "innocuous methods" of contraception.[37]

Meanwhile Freud was becoming more conscious of, or at least more explicit in his love for Fliess. He told Martha's sister, Minna, "He is a most unusual person, good nature personified: and I believe, if it came to it, he would for all his genius, be goodness itself. Therefore his sunlike clarity, his pluck".[38] He began addressing Fliess as "My beloved friend", and, in the same letter, told him that Martha had unexpectedly joined him on holiday, thereby putting a stop to their planned meeting in Csorba. To this he added that Martha was "coming back to life again" now she did "not have to expect a child for a year because we are now living in abstinence", adding, "you know the reasons for this as well".[39]

Soon after Freud completed another essay about hysteria. In it he rejected Pierre Janet's attribution of the self-division involved to congenital mental weakness. Rather, Freud said, this division is caused by "an act of will on the part of the patient".[40] Whether this eventuates in hysteria depends on whether the feelings against which patients assert their will can be converted into bodily symptoms. If this is not possible the feelings may be displaced or projected onto a more acceptable idea, which then becomes the focus of obsessional rather than hysterical symptoms. In either case treatment entails redirecting the patient's attention to the divided off – repressed or projected – feelings causing their symptoms, feelings which Freud now regarded as always connected with the patient's love life.

In this Freud began taking issue with Breuer. It left him isolated. In May 1894 he told Fliess:

> You are the only other, the *alter* . . . I am pretty much alone here in the elucidation of the neuroses. They look upon me as pretty much of a monomaniac, while I have the distinct feeling that I have touched upon one of the great secrets of nature.[41]

He spelt out these "great secrets" further in an essay published in January 1895. In it he wrote of defence against unacceptable feelings and ideas resulting in

---

[36] Jones 1961 pp. 215–6.

[37] Draft B. The etiology of the neuroses, to Fliess, 8 February 1893, in Masson pp. 39–44, 44.

[38] To Minna Bernays, 7 April 1893, in Masson p. 2.

[39] To Fliess, 20 August 1893, ibid. pp. 53, 54.

[40] S. Freud (1894) The neuro-psychoses of defence, SE3 pp. 45–61, 46.

[41] To Fliess, 21 May 1894, in Masson pp. 73, 74.

phobic anxiety against which patients may further defend themselves by developing a "substitutive obsession".[42] Later he related this to religion, but not until some time after his involvement with Fliess was over.

He was now more concerned with dreams. Just as he had written about them in his love letters to Martha, he now wrote about them to Fliess. Illustrating their wish-fulfilling character he told him a dream of Breuer's nephew Rudi, who, like them, was also a doctor:

> [He] is a late riser. He has his maidservant wake him, and then is very reluctant to obey her. One morning she woke him again and, since he did not want to listen to her, called him by his name, "Mr.Rudi". Thereupon the sleeper hallucinated a hospital chart (compare the Fudolfinerhaus) with the name "Rudolf Kaufmann" on it and said to himself, "So R.K. is already in the hospital; then I do not need to go there", and went on sleeping![43]

The next month Freud sent Fliess proofs of the book he had written with Breuer. In it he concluded by tentatively rejecting Breuer's hypnoid theory of hysteria in favour of the argument that in all hysteria "the primary factor is defence".[44] Disagreeing with Breuer, he became increasingly preoccupied with Fliess, about whom he dreamt in a dream that became central in formulating his theory of the unconscious. The dream occurred on the night of 23–24 July 1895. Interpreting its central motif – a drug called "trimethylamin" – Freud wrote:

> Trimethylamin was an allusion not only to the immensely powerful factor of sexuality, but also to a person whose agreement I recalled whenever I felt isolated in my opinions. Surely this friend who played so large a part in my life must appear again in these trains of thought.[45]

His friend did indeed appear in his associations to his dream. Furthermore, the next day, without mentioning the dream to Fliess, Freud chivvied him:

> Daimonie [Demon], why don't you write? How are you? Don't you care at all any more about what I am doing? . . . Are we friends only in misfortune? Or do we also want to share the experiences of calm times with each other? Where will you spend the month of August?[46]

Freud himself spent that August in Venice. "Carissimo Guglielmo", he wrote, telling him he was "looking forward tremendously" to seeing him soon in Berlin.[47] Inspired by meeting with him there, he excitedly started writing a draft

42 S. Freud (1895) Obsessions and phobias, **SE3** pp. 74–82, 82.

43 To Fliess, 4 March 1895, in Masson p. 114.

44 In Freud and Breuer p. 286.

45 S. Freud (1900) *The Interpretation of Dreams*, **SE4 and 5** p. 117.

46 To Fliess, 24 July 1895, in Masson p. 134.

47 To Fliess, 28 August 1895, ibid. p. 136.

of his newly developing theory (of psychology, psychopathology, and wishful- and reality-based unconscious and conscious thinking, and free association)[48] on the train home. He sent the resulting pages to Fliess, saying "I scribbled them full at one stretch since my return". To this he added that he was retaining a third notebook and ended, apropos their recent meeting, "My yearning for you and your company this time came somewhat later, but was very great".[49]

Perhaps Freud's yearning for Fliess contributed to his writing in his note- books about the longing of babies for their mothers in their absence. He described this longing as impelling what he called the baby's first "primary process" thinking, his imagining, hallucinating, and dreaming that his mother is there. Putting this in neurological terms, Freud wrote:

> Let us suppose, for instance, that the mnemic image wished for [by the baby] is the image of the mother's breast . . . The aim is to go back to the missing neurone b and to release the sensation of identity.[50]

Of these and other insights inspired by Fliess, Freud told him:

> The barriers suddenly lifted, the veils dropped, and everything became transparent – from the details of the neuroses to the determinants of consciousness. . . . the primary and secondary processes . . . attention and defense . . . the sexual determination of repression . . . I can scarcely manage to contain my delight.[51]

In early December a newspaper welcomed Freud's book with Breuer as "surgery of the soul".[52] The next day Freud's sixth and last child was born:

> Dearest Wilhelm, If it had been a son, I would have sent you the news by telegram, because he would have carried your name. Since it turned out to be a little daughter by the name of Anna, she is being introduced to you belatedly. Today at 3 : 15 she pushed her way into my consulting hour.[53]

More exciting, it seemed, to Freud was Fliess. Five days later he wrote to him of his joy at getting a letter from him. It enabled him, he said, to forget his "lone- liness and privation",[54] adding in the new year:

> How much I owe you: solace, understanding, stimulation in my loneliness, meaning to my life that I gained through you, and finally even health that no one else could have given back to me.[55]

---

[48] S. Freud (1895) Project for a scientific psychology, **SE1** pp. 295–387.

[49] To Fliess, 8 October 1895, in Masson p. 141.

[50] Freud 1895 p. 329.

[51] To Fliess, 20 October 1895, in Masson p. 146.

[52] In Jones 1961 p. 224.

[53] To Fliess, 3 December 1895, in Masson p. 153.

[54] To Fliess, 8 December 1895, ibid. p. 154.

[55] To Fliess, 1 January 1896, ibid. p. 158.

He included an essay about feelings of conflict, self-reproach, mortification, and mourning, and about their defensive form in hysteria, obsessional neurosis, paranoia, and what he called "acute hallucinatory amentia".[56]

The next month he sent off two essays for publication. In one he described his method for the first time as "psycho-analysis".[57] In the other he announced that obsessional ideas – to which, as I have said, he later likened religion – are a defence against the truth of love and sex. They are, he said, "invariably trans-formed self-reproaches which have re-emerged from repression and which always relate to some sexual act that was performed with pleasure in childhood".[58]

Previously he had written to Fliess linking hysteria with sexual "abuse".[59] Now he made this idea public. In a lecture that April he argued that hysteria is due to the patient repressing from consciousness the truth of having been sexually "seduced" when he or she was 3 or 4. With the awakening of sexuality in adolescence, he said, the memory of this event presses for expression. But since it is repressed it cannot be expressed consciously. It can only be expressed unconsciously in bodily or hysterical form.[60] Hence the patient's symptoms. Freud's lecture to this effect was greeted with an "icy reception", he told Fliess.[61] "I am as isolated as you would wish me to be", he added a few days later, "a void is forming all around me".[62]

He was now prevented from seeing Fliess by his father becoming very ill.

> To meet you in Berlin, to hear about the new magic from you for a few hours, and then suddenly to have to rush back during the day or night because of news which might turn out to be a false alarm – that is something I really want to avoid, and to this fear I sacrifice the burning desire once again to live fully, with head and heart simultaneously, to be a *zoon politikon* [social animal], and, moreover, to see you.[63]

Three months later Freud's father died, on 23 October 1896. Soon after, fol-lowing the death of her fiancé, Ignaz Schönberg, Freud's sister-in-law, Minna, came to live with the Freuds in Vienna.

....

56 Draft K. The neuroses of defence, to Fliess, 1 January 1896, ibid. pp. 162–70.

57 S. Freud (1896a) Heredity and the aetiology of the neuroses, **SE3** pp. 143–56, 151.

58 S. Freud (1896) Further remarks on the neuro-psychoses of defence, **SE3** pp. 162–85, 169.

59 To Fliess, 30 May 1893, in Masson p. 49.

60 S. Freud (1896) The aetiology of hysteria, **SE3** pp. 191–221.

61 To Fliess, 26 April 1896, in Masson p. 184.

62 To Fliess, 4 May 1896, ibid. p. 185.

63 To Fliess, 15 July 1896, ibid. p. 194.

Freud now became increasingly preoccupied with dreams of love and sex, which he recounted to Fliess, as in the following example:

> I was going up a staircase with very few clothes on. I was moving, as the dream explicitly emphasized, with great agility. (My heart – reassurance!) Suddenly I noticed, however, that a woman was coming after me, and thereupon set the sensation, so common in dreams, of being glued to the spot, of being paralyzed. The accompanying feeling was not anxiety but erotic excitement.[64]

He wrote of his defences. He connected them with Fliess: "Something from the deepest depths of my own neurosis set itself against any advance in the understanding of the neuroses", he wrote to him, "and you have somehow been involved in it".[65]

A couple of months later he confided that he had abandoned his "*neurotica*", his seduction theory of hysteria.[66] He now became increasingly interested in dreams. His associations to them, perhaps prompted by love of Fliess, reminded him of his first initiation into sex and religion by his Catholic nursemaid in Freiberg, "an ugly, elderly, but clever woman, who told me a great deal about God Almighty and hell". His dreams also reminded him of his first sexual desire for his mother, spending the night with her, and doubtless seeing her "*nudam*" on the train taking the family from Leipzig to Vienna when he was 2.[67] This in turn led Freud to tell Fliess his nascent Oedipus complex theory of sex and love:

> I have found, in my own case too, [the phenomenon of] being in love with my mother and jealous of my father, and I now consider it a universal event in early childhood . . . we can [thus] understand the gripping power of *Oedipus Rex* . . . [everyone] in the audience was once a budding Oedipus in fantasy and each recoils in horror from the dream fulfillment here transplanted into reality.[68]

Impatient for Fliess to reply, Freud described to him his changing moods:

> Like the landscapes seen by a traveller from a train . . . days when I drag myself about dejected because I have understood nothing . . . and then again days when a flash of lightning illuminates the interrelations.[69]

Illuminations included dawning understanding of mental illness being shaped, as he told Fliess,[70] by the developmental stage – oral, anal, or genital,

---

64 To Fliess, 31 May 1897, ibid. p. 249.

65 To Fliess, 7 July 1897, ibid. p. 255.

66 To Fliess, 21 September 1897, ibid. p. 264.

67 To Fliess, 3 October 1897, ibid. p. 268.

68 To Fliess, 15 October 1897, ibid. p. 272.

69 To Fliess, 27 October 1897, ibid. p. 274.

70 To Fliess 14 March 1897, ibid. pp. 280–1.

as Freud put it – when the repression of the patient's love life first begins. Early the next year he completed an essay which put this theory into print.[71]

To undo the defences against love and sex, which he now believed to be the source of neurosis, Freud abandoned hypnosis for free association which he had theorized in terms of free-flowing wishful-thinking in the notes inspired by his meeting with Fliess in September 1895.[72] Hypnosis, he said, all too often awakens the patient's love for the therapist. It had done so in the case of Breuer's patient Anna O. The same happened to Freud. "One day", he wrote, "one of my most acquiescent patients, with whom hypnotism had enabled me to bring about the most marvellous results . . . woke up on one occasion [and] threw her arms round my neck".[73] Whatever beneficial effects hypnosis might have, they were lost when the "personal relation" between the therapist and patient was disturbed by, for instance, the patient's therapy ending.[74]

Free association initially seemed to solve the problem. Freud called it the "main" rule of psychoanalysis, requiring "the patient to say whatever he likes".[75] He also called it "the fundamental rule of psycho-analysis", telling the patient "whatever comes into one's head must be reported without criticizing it".[76] In dream interpretation, he said, it involves:

> Abandoning all those purposive ideas which normally govern our reflections, in focusing our attention on a single element of the dream and in then taking note of whatever involuntary thoughts may occur in connection with it.[77]

Freud continued to be inspired by Fliess. Telling him he was "deep in the dream book",[78] he also told him, "I am so immensely glad that you are giving me the gift of the Other . . . I cannot write entirely without an audience, but do not at all mind writing only for you".[79] Another time, after they again met, he wrote:

> Here I live in ill humor and in darkness until you come; I get things off my chest; rekindle my flickering flame at your steadfast one and feel well again; and after your departure, I again have been given eyes to see, and what I see is beautiful and good.[80]

[71] S. Freud (1898) Sexuality in the aetiology of the neuroses, SE3 pp. 263–85.

[72] See especially Part III, 5 October 1895, SE1 p. 376 n. 1.

[73] Freud 1925 p. 27.

[74] Ibid. p. 27.

[75] S. Freud (1910) Five lectures on psycho-analysis, SE11 pp. 7–55, 33.

[76] S. Freud (1912) The dynamics of transference, SE12 pp. 99–108, 107.

[77] Freud 1900 pp. 526–7.

[78] To Fliess, 9 February 1898, in Masson p. 298.

[79] To Fliess, 18 May 1898, ibid. p. 313.

[80] To Fliess, 4 January 1899, ibid. p. 339.

Love of Fliess, it seems, reminded him of his first love. He told him about his essay, "Screen memories".[81] In the essay he wrote of his teenage love, on revisiting Freiberg, for the daughter of a wool merchant friend of his father there.

> It was my first calf-love and sufficiently intense, but I kept it completely secret. After a few days the girl [Gisela] went off to her school . . . and it was this separation . . . that brought my longings to a really high pitch. I passed many hours in solitary walks through the lovely woods that I had found once more and spent my time building castles in the air.[82]

Now it was Fliess, not his first love, who preoccupied him: "I cannot do without you", he wrote, "as the representative of the Other".[83] And then, at the end of the year, 1899, his dream book was finished. It famously ended with his announcing that interpreting dreams is "the royal road to a knowledge of the unconscious".[84] Dream interpretation, it turned out, might open the door that William James complained closed him off from religious and mystical experience. Freud, by contrast, regarded opening this door – repression – as means of discovering the full truth of our feelings of sex and love. Dream interpretation, he said, entails undoing the "dream-work" censorship disguising unconscious wishes through what Freud called "condensation", "displacement", "visual presentation", and "secondary revision".

But why do we defend against love and sex? It was with this question that Freud now became preoccupied. He anticipated to Fliess that a "theory of sexuality may be the immediate successor to the dream book".[85] Three months later he reported, "New ideas come slowly, but there never is total stillness . . . I am collecting material for the sexual theory and am waiting for a spark to set the accumulated material on fire".[86] He was still waiting, it seems, that summer when, writing to Fliess of his holiday home in Bellevue, on the outskirts of Vienna, he speculated:

> Do you suppose that someday one will read on a marble tablet on this house: Here, on July 24, 1895, the secret of the dream revealed itself to Dr. Sigm. Freud. So far there is little prospect of it.[87]

---

[81] To Fliess, 25 May 1899, ibid. p. 351.

[82] S. Freud (1899) Screen memories, SE3 pp. 303–22, 313.

[83] To Fliess, 21 September 1899, in Masson p. 374.

[84] Freud 1900 p. 608.

[85] To Fliess, 11 October 1899, in Masson p. 379.

[86] To Fliess, 26 January 1900, ibid. p. 397.

[87] To Fliess, 12 June 1900, ibid. p. 417.

Freud's further discoveries would have to be made without Fliess. That August they met at the Achesee, near Innsbruck, quarrelled, and never met again. Freud tried to patch things up but Fliess was too aggrieved. He became convinced that Freud had given away his theories about bisexuality to a young man, Otto Weininger, and with a letter about this grievance,[88] their correspondence ended.

Therapy and religion

Freud now applied what he had learnt during his love affair with Fliess to both psychoanalysis and religion. Replying in a lecture in December 1904 to the charge that his method of therapy was a species of "modern mysticism",[89] he differentiated his method from hypnosis. He likened the difference to a distinction made by Leonardo da Vinci between the artist putting on paint where there was none before and the sculptor taking away from stone all that hides a statue within it. Psychoanalysis conforms to the latter method. It involves revealing what Pierre Janet called "an unconscious *idée fixe*".[90] But, since uncovering such ideas is unpleasurable, psychoanalysis entails re-educating patients to overcome their defences against them. Furthermore, since these defences come from "aversion from sexuality" – from the patient's "incapacity for loving" – the doctor also has to overcome his own defences including the "prurience and prudery" besetting sex.[91]

Yet sex's origins are entirely innocent. Writing of its developmental beginning, Freud noted

> No one who has seen a baby sinking back satiated from the breast and falling asleep with flushed cheeks and a blissful smile . . . can escape the reflection that this picture persists as a prototype of the expression of sexual satisfaction in later life.[92]

He also described the pleasure children derive from stimulating their anus and genitals. Its first object is the person the child most loves. But then "disgust, feelings of shame and the claims of aesthetic and moral ideals" result in these sources of pleasure being repressed.[93] They only re-emerge with puberty, when they are again liable to defensive repression in so far as their object is incestuous.

---

88 To Fliess, 27 July 1904, ibid. p. 466–8.

89 S. Freud (1905) On psychotherapy, **SE7** pp. 257–68, 258.

90 Ibid. p. 266.

91 Ibid. p. 267.

92 S. Freud (1905d) *Three Essays on the Theory of Sexuality*, **SE7** p. 182.

93 Ibid. p. 177.

An example was an 18-year-old patient, Dora. Freud described how, awakened to sexual love by a friend of the family, Herr K, Dora was driven to defend against it by returning to her childhood love of her father which, in repressed form, was expressed in a nervous cough and anorexia. Their treatment, said Freud, depended on bringing Dora's repressed love to consciousness. But, before her symptoms could be relieved, Dora quit therapy. She thereby taught Freud that, just as hypnosis arouses the patient's love and defences against love in relation to the therapist, so too does psychoanalysis. Freud accordingly concluded that, to be effective, psychoanalysis must put into words and thereby help make more conscious what he called the patient's unconscious "transference" of their love and its repression into therapy. The transference, he said, proves that therapy is above all about love. Or, as he put it to Jung "Essentially, one might say, the cure is effected by love. And actually transference provides the most cogent, indeed the only unassailable proof that neuroses are determined by the individual's love life".[94]

As long as the patient's transference-love for the analyst is not put into words its therapeutic effect is akin to cure through religious faith as in places where "a miracle-working image is worshipped, or where a holy or divine personage has revealed himself to men and has promised them relief from their suffering in return for their worship".[95] He dwelt more on religion in an essay written in February 1907. In it he argued that religious rituals are a compulsive defence aimed at keeping guilt-evoking feelings about sex and love unconscious. They are like obsessional symptoms, as in the following example.

> A girl whom I was able to observe was under a compulsion to rinse round her washbasin several times after washing. The significance of this ceremonial action lay in the proverbial saying: "Don't throw away dirty water till you have clean". Her action was intended to give a warning to her sister, of whom she was very fond, and to restrain her from getting divorced from her unsatisfactory husband until she had established a relationship with a better man.[96]

He went on to argue that the "pious observances . . . prayers, invocations, etc". of those who call themselves "miserable sinners" function similarly as "defensive or protective measures".[97] In both obsessional and religious rituals, he concluded, psychical energy is repressed and displaced into meticulous execution of the ritual involved.

---

[94] To Jung, 6 December 1906, in W. McGuire (1974) *The Freud/Jung Letters*, London: Hogarth, pp. 12–3.

[95] S. Freud (1905) Psychical (or mental) treatment, **SE7** pp. 283–302, 289.

[96] S. Freud (1907) Obsessive actions and religious practices, **SE9** pp. 117–27, 120.

[97] Ibid. p. 124.

Psychoanalysis, by contrast, seeks to free people from all such defensive repression. Religion – Christianity, at least – rewards repression with the promise of heaven to come. Psychoanalysis makes no such promises. Explaining this to a Protestant pastor from Zurich, Oskar Pfister, with whom Freud became close friends, he wrote:

> Our public, no matter of what racial origin, is irreligious, we are generally thoroughly irreligious ourselves and, as the other ways of sublimation which *we* substitute for religion are too difficult for most patients, our treatment generally results in the seeking out of satisfaction. On top of this there is the fact that we are unable to see anything forbidden or sinful in sexual satisfaction, but regard it as a valuable part of human experience. You are aware that for us the term "sex" includes what you in your pastoral work call love, and is certainly not restricted to the crude pleasure of the senses. Thus our patients have to find in humanity what we are unable to promise them from above and are unable to supply them with ourselves. Things are therefore much more difficult for us, and in the resolution of the transference many of our successes come to grief.[98]

The same year, 1909, a case by Freud bearing on religion and obsessional neurosis was published. It involved a 29-year-old man, now known as the Rat Man, who came for treatment on account of a crippling obsession that, if he did not repay a debt, which he had in fact repaid, his father and girlfriend would be subjected to an eastern torture in which a basin of rats is inverted on the victim's buttocks so as to gnaw into his or her anus. In dwelling on dread of those he loved being thus punished, the Rat Man also dwelt on religious threats of punishment in this life and in hell to come. Fearing such punishment – and particularly fearing lest thinking about sex and love kill his father – he had repressed such thoughts as a child and instead tried to pray. But he kept finding unwanted thoughts intruding. If, for instance, he said, "May God protect him", he would find an "evil spirit" insinuating the word "not".[99] Nevertheless he became "devoutly religious" as a teenager, and only later became a "free thinker".[100]

Subsequently, however, his earlier defences returned and with them, his obsessive symptoms. With these symptoms also returned his earlier mixed feelings of love and hate for God and for his father. He transferred these feelings into his treatment with Freud. He imagined in his dreams and waking fantasies heaping filthy abuse on Freud and his family despite outwardly

---

[98] To Pfister, 9 February 1909, in H. Meng & E. Freud (1963) *Psychoanalysis and Faith: The Letters of Sigmund Freud and Oskar Pfister*, London: Hogarth, pp. 16–7.

[99] S. Freud (1909) Notes upon a case of obsessional neurosis, **SE10** pp. 155–249, 193.

[100] Ibid. p. 169.

according him the utmost respect. He wondered out loud how Freud could let himself be so abused. At this he would get off the couch in case, lying near him, Freud might beat him as his father had when he was a child.

The success of his treatment, it seems, depended on both his love and hate being put into words. Writing more generally, Freud told Pfister, "I have, as you admit, done a great deal for love, but experience does not confirm that it lies at the base of everything, unless, as is psychologically correct, hate is included with it".[101] In this Freud was akin to William James, who criticized mind-cure and Christian Science therapy for focusing on what is good to the neglect of what is bad. Unlike James, however, Freud deplored religion. He denounced "the powerful religious inhibition of thought . . . brought into play by education".[102] Previously, he argued, the sexual organs were "worshipped as gods" and "the divine nature of their functions" was transmitted "to all newly learned human activities". Subsequently, however, "so much of the divine and sacred was ultimately extracted from sexuality . . . the exhausted remnant fell into contempt".[103] Instead people came to look to God and religion not as means to love and sex but as defence against them, as also occurs, he said, in the "parental complex" of early childhood.[104]

Some defend against love and sex with repression. Others defend with paranoia. Fliess had done just this in his final imagined grievances against Freud regarding Otto Weininger. Or so Freud claimed. He told Jung, "My erstwhile friend Fliess developed a beautiful paranoia after he had disposed of his inclination, certainly not slight, toward me".[105] As for his own defence against love of Fliess, he told the Hungarian psychoanalyst, Sandor Ferenczi:

> I *no longer* have any need to uncover my personality completely . . . Since Fliess's case, with the overcoming of which you recently saw me occupied, that need has been extinguished. A part of homosexual cathexis has been withdrawn and made use of to enlarge my own ego. I have succeeded where the paranoiac fails.[106]

To this he added a few days later:

> You probably imagine that I have secrets quite other than those I have reserved for myself, or you believe that my secrets are connected with a special sorrow, whereas

---

[101] To Pfister, 17 March 1910, in Meng and Freud p. 36.

[102] S. Freud (1910) *Leonardo da Vinci and a Memory of his Childhood*, **SE**11 pp. 63–157, 79.

[103] Ibid. p. 97.

[104] Ibid. p. 123.

[105] To Jung, 17 February 1908, in McGuire p. 134.

[106] To Ferenczi, 6 October 1910, in E. Jones (1958) *Sigmund Freud: Life and Work, Vol. II*, London: Hogarth, p. 92.

> I feel capable of handling everything and am pleased with the greater independence that results from having overcome my homosexuality.[107]

In his published writing Freud dwelt on bisexuality in hysteria,[108] and in psychosis, which he also related to religion. He described, for instance, the autobiographical account of a middle-aged judge, Daniel Paul Schreber, of his paranoid schizophrenic breakdown. It included Schreber imagining himself becoming a woman and being sexually attacked, penetrated, and controlled by God. Freud interpreted this delusion as fulfilling Schreber's sexual love for his father as a child through projecting it onto God, and, in hospital, onto his doctor, Fleschsig. At the same time Schreber also glorified himself as repository of God's sexual love. The hospital report on him noted:

> The culminating point of the patient's delusional system is his belief that he has a mission to redeem the world, and to restore mankind to their lost state of bliss. He was called to this task, so he asserts, by direct inspiration from God . . . He has a feeling that enormous numbers of "female nerves" have already passed over into his body, and out of them a new race will proceed, through a process of direct impregnation by God.[109]

He even imagined not only that he was penetrated by God but that he was one with Him, that he was God himself. This, he said, was proved by his being able to look into the sun without being dazzled by it.

Freud criticized his sometime colleague, Alfred Adler, as similarly bombastic. He described him as forgetting love in favour of God-like grandiosity in creating what he described as "a world system without love".[110] As for his earlier love for Fliess, said Freud, in mentioning him for the last time, he had "overcome" it.[111]

Freud nevertheless remained convinced that love is at the heart of therapy. Just as, he said, Schreber transferred love and sex from his father onto God and onto his psychiatrist, Fleschsig, so too, he argued, patients generally transfer their love, and defences against love, onto the psychoanalyst. Their "transference-love" is both a source of resistance and also an ally. For it makes the patients' otherwise repressed and unconscious longings "immediate and manifest".[112] Religion, by

---

[107] To Ferenczi, 17 October 1910, in Masson p. 4 n. 3.

[108] S. Freud (1908) Hysterical phantasies and their relation to bisexuality, **SE9** pp. 159–66.

[109] S. Freud (1911) Psycho-analytic notes on an autobiographical account of a case of paranoia (*dementia paranoides*), **SE12** pp. 9–79, 16–17.

[110] To Pfister, 26 February 1911, in Meng and Freud p. 48.

[111] To Ferenczi, 16 December 1911, in Masson p. 4 n. 3.

[112] S. Freud (1912) The dynamics of transference, **SE12** pp. 99–108, 108.

contrast, does the reverse: it shores up women's and men's defences against sex and love. Or so Freud claimed, criticizing "the ascetic current in Christianity" whereby monks become "entirely occupied with the struggle against libidinal temptation",[113] thereby reinforcing an already prevalent tendency whereby we divide sex from love for fear lest together they lead to incest, as they would were we to have sex with those we first love – our parents.

To free patients from their resulting defences against sex, wrote Freud, analysts must free themselves from similar defences in themselves through adopting a method similar to the free association he recommended to his patients. The analyst, he said, should adopt a non-directive attitude, free from all defensive selection and bias "maintaining the same 'evenly-suspended attention' (as I have called it) in the face of all one hears".[114] Or, as he also put it, the analyst "must turn his own unconscious like a receptive organ towards the transmitting unconscious of the patient" so as to remain free of all impurity, distortion, and resistance.[115]

Religion stops any such freedom, said Freud. Its practices both express unconscious wishes concerning love and sex and in doing so form a rigid defence against them. Freud detailed this in a book, *Totem and Taboo*, arguably inspired by love of Jung, as his dream book had been inspired by love of Fliess. But whereas the dream book documents Freud's pursuit of the truth regarding the unconscious, *Totem and Taboo* is an often rather dreary imposition of Freud's preconceived theories about psychoanalysis onto religion, showing scant regard for the truth of its history.

Having discovered from his own self-analysis, and from the analysis of others, the adult repercussions of repressed sexual love for the mother, and wish to kill the father on this account, Freud projected this into religion. He argued that in human prehistory brothers banded together to kill the patriarchal leader of their clan. Guilt about this, Freud went on, survives in the ritual totem meal of clan societies. It involves, he said, displacing onto the totem animal of the clan the wish to kill and eat the father. The totem meal both expresses and atones for the realization of this wish, as do the rules of a clan against marrying fellow clan members, originally those set free by the sons of its patriarchal leader. Eventually, Freud went on, the longing of sons for their father resulted in their creating gods. Animals lost their sacred character. They

[113] S. Freud (1912) On the universal tendency to debasement in the sphere of love, **SE11** pp. 179–90, 188.

[114] S. Freud (1912) Recommendations to physicians practising psycho-analysis, **SE12** pp. 111–20, 111–2.

[115] Ibid. p. 115.

were offered to the gods as a sacrifice. In Christianity the son of God sacrificed himself. The Eucharist repeats this act. It is similar to totemism except that totemism, unlike the Eucharist or Mass, repeats an actual deed, insisted Freud, the actual killing of the father in man's prehistory.

Freud's account of the history of religion in this respect is extremely far-fetched. Less far-fetched is his account of the ramifications of religion in individual psychology, as in the Rat Man and Schreber cases. Another example, now known as the Wolf Man, involved a Russian who came for analysis with Freud when he was 23. His symptoms included impotence and failure in both love and work. In analysis with Freud it transpired that these symptoms originated in childhood anxiety, starting when he was 4, lest were he to realize his longing to make love with his father he would have to become like his mother and have no penis like her. He was so anxious as a child that his mother sought to calm him down with Bible stories. He also sought to calm himself with various religious rituals. Before going to bed he kissed all the holy pictures in his room, recited prayers, and made numerous signs of the cross before going to sleep.

Born on Christmas Day, he imagined he was Christ submitting to God the Father. When he was 10, however, this gave way to his submitting to a German tutor. Because the tutor was an atheist this entailed giving up his previous religious piety. All that remained was a scatological obsession – "having to think of the Holy Trinity whenever he saw three heaps of dung lying together in the road".[116] In analysis he transferred onto Freud his previous submissiveness to God and others. Still feeling the need to tear himself away from submission to Freud, he returned for further analysis during the war and was thereby relieved, apparently, of this "piece of transference".[117]

Whereas the Wolf Man vacillated in his religious belief, Freud remained a staunch non-believer. "Incidentally", he once asked Pfister, "why was it that none of all the pious ever discovered psycho-analysis? Why did it have to wait for a completely godless Jew?"[118] Pfister sought to reassure him, "you are not godless, for he who lives the truth lives in God, and he who strives for the freeing of love 'dwelleth in God' ".[119] For Freud, freeing love now included analyzing several of his patients' defensive masturbatory incantations.[120] More often, however, during and after the war, he dwelt on loss and death.

---

[116] S. Freud (1918) From the history of an infantile neurosis, SE17, pp. 7–122, 68.

[117] Ibid. p. 122.

[118] To Pfister, 9 October 1918, in Meng and Freud p. 63.

[119] To Freud, 29 October 1918, in Meng and Freud p. 63.

[120] S. Freud (1919) A child is being beaten, SE17 pp. 179–204.

Loss, mysticism, and death

Disappointment in his love of Fliess, and then of Jung, together with the losses of the war, perhaps contributed to Freud shifting his attention, during the war, from defences of repression and projection of love and sex to the defence of identification or "introjection". He now dwelt on ways people may deal with disappointment in, or death of, those they love by imagining they are one with them as an ideal figure in the unconscious.[121] After the war, preoccupied with the suffering of shell-shock victims, and the sudden death of his daughter, Sophie, on 25 January 1920, in that year's flu epidemic, Freud further revised his theory of the unconscious. Previously he had regarded it as constituted by wish-fulfilling dreams of love and sex. Now he attended to its nightmares. He described them as driven by a compulsion to repeat trauma (traumas of war and of separation and loss, for instance) in the hope of thereby abolishing the anxieties involved. This "repetition compulsion", he said, seeks to reduce stimulation to zero, as when we are dead. He accordingly described this compulsion as driven by "the death instinct". He likened it to the feigning of death to overcome the fears it arouses involved in the "Nirvana principle",[122] now defined in Buddhism as "Extinction; blowing out: like extinction of self which brings enlightenment and liberation from pain".[123]

Freud was no Buddhist. But he now likened his method of free association to mystical contemplation. He likened it to the method recommended by the Swedenborgian mystic, Garth Wilkinson (after whom William James' younger brother had been called). Quoting Wilkinson, Freud wrote that his method entailed leaving aside reason and the will and trusting to "an influx" whereby the faculties of the mind are "directed to ends they know not of".[124]

Opening oneself to whatever comes arguably depends on love and trust in others. Whereas William James said nothing of this in his account of self-surrender to religious experience as therapy, Freud very much emphasized love in his account of therapy. Appreciating this, his pastor friend, Pfister, linked his work with that of Plato:

> I have made a wonderful discovery in Plato which will give you pleasure. . . . Plato wrote the following: "For the art of healing . . . is knowledge of the body's loves . . . and he who is able to distinguish between the good and bad kinds, and is able to bring about a change, so that the body acquires one kind of love instead of the

---

121 S. Freud (1917) Mourning and melancholia, **SE14** pp. 243–58.

122 S. Freud (1920) *Beyond the Pleasure Principle*, **SE18** pp. 7–64, 56.

123 K. Armstrong (2000) *Buddha*, London: Weidenfeld & Nicolson, p. 186.

124 S. Freud (1920) A note on the prehistory of the technique of analysis, **SE18** pp. 263–5, 264.

other, and is able to impart love to those in whom there is none . . . is the best physician".[125]

Whilst Pfister thus emphasized love in therapy, Freud now described it in religion. He described fellow-Christians identifying with each other in love of Christ with whom, he said, they identify as an ideal version of themselves. Similarly, he said, the lover identifies with his beloved in being in love. But, he argued, this oneness with another is an illusion. The lover, said Freud, makes his beloved the imagined locus of all he most idealizes, loves, and holds dear in himself. When we are in love, Freud wrote, "the ego becomes more and more unassuming and modest, and the object more and more sublime and precious".[126] The beloved, he said, consumes the lover's ego.

Being in love is akin to hypnosis. It involves "the same humble subjection, the same compliance, the same absence of criticism, towards the hypnotist as towards the loved object".[127] Nevertheless he advocated the same absence of criticism in the psychoanalyst towards his patients. In an article written in the summer of 1922 he continued to advise:

> The analytic physician . . . to avoid so far as possible reflection and the construction of conscious expectations, not to try to fix anything that he heard particularly in his memory, and by these means to catch the drift of the patient's unconscious with his own unconscious.[128]

By now, as I have said, he was mindful of the unconscious as constituted by nightmares as well as by pleasurable dreams of love and sex. In the last months of 1922 he recounted these nightmares in terms of a reported case of what he called "demonological neurosis".[129] The case involved an artist who, despairing of his painting being any good, made a pact with the devil to help him. A month before the pact fell due he was seized with terrible convulsions in church. Only the mother of God could save him, a belief Freud analyzed as the artist's defence against dread of his father.

Freud now theorized this defence more generally. He described all children as defending against love and dread of the father, in rivalry with him for sexual love of the mother, by introjecting and identifying with him as an ideal superego inside them. Personalizing, in paternal terms, the defences of the ego against love and sex, Freud now referred to the latter as an effect of instincts

[125] To Freud, 14 January 1921, in Meng and Freud p. 80.

[126] S. Freud (1921) *Group Psychology and the Analysis of the Ego*, **SE18** pp. 69–143, 113.

[127] Ibid. p. 114.

[128] S. Freud (1923) Two encyclopaedia articles, **SE18** pp. 235–59, 239.

[129] S. Freud (1923) A seventeenth-century demonological neurosis, **SE19** pp. 72–105.

within what he called the "id". Jung equated the superego with God as an archetype in the collective unconscious. Not so Pfister. In July 1923 he told Freud:

> I have completely finished with the Jungian manner. Those high-falutin interpretations which proclaim every kind of muck to be spiritual jam of a high order and try to smuggle a minor Apollo or Christ into every corked-up little mind simply will not do. It is Hegelianism transferred to psychology; everything that is must be reasonable. If only that theory were true![130]

Freud's correspondents now included the then celebrated French writer, Romain Rolland. Freud wrote to him, as he had to many others before, about love. He told him that he was "a disciple of the love of mankind", that love was as essential "to the survival of the human race" as technology and science.[131] He foccused more on this in an open letter, as it were, to Pfister about religion. In it he dwelt, as William James had in his book, *The Varieties of Religious Experience*, not so much on organized religion as on individual religious experience. Unlike James, however, Freud argued that this experience is false.

Forgetting his previous insights about the truth of psychical reality – of fantasy – including imagination and dreaming – he dismissed religious experience on this account as an illusion. He argued that it is founded on imagining and believing that goodness and justice inhere in God. Some claim, he said, that this belief is founded in "divine revelation".[132] But this is no ground for belief: "If one man has gained an unshakable conviction of the true reality of religious doctrines from a state of ecstasy which has deeply moved him, of what significance is that to others?"[133] William James argued something similar.

Freud, however, went further. He maintained that religious experience is a defensive retreat to infancy. Imagining goodness and justice inhering in God, he said, stems from an infantile wish that the first object of our love and desire – our mothers – will protect us from all danger. Religious experience, he said, also stems from transferring this wish onto our fathers whom, as children, we also dread and seek to propitiate.

Unlike the ideas of science, religious ideas cannot be proved through experience. Nor, Freud went on, can spiritualism prove the existence of an afterlife. For spiritualist mediums cannot demonstrate that the appearance and utterances of spirits in their trances are not merely the products of their imagination. By contrast, he maintained, psychoanalysis seeks to restore its patients to reality

---

[130] To Freud, 19 July 1922, in Meng and Freud pp. 86–7.

[131] To Rolland, 26 January 1926, in S. Freud (1926a) To Romain Rolland, **SE20** p. 279.

[132] S. Freud (1927) *The Future of an Illusion*, **SE21** pp. 5–56, 21.

[133] Ibid. p. 28.

and reason. Religion might seek to evade the challenge of science through affirming "belief in a higher spiritual being, whose qualities are indefinable and whose purposes cannot be discerned". But religion thereby loses all claim to "human interest".[134] Better far, he insisted, is science. It is no illusion. But it would be an illusion, he concluded, "to suppose that what science cannot give us we can get elsewhere".[135]

Pfister dissented.[136] Against him Freud argued that psychoanalysis necessarily entails rejecting religion. Nor is the analyst an ersatz God. "[H]owever warm-heartedly the analyst may behave", Freud told Pfister, "he cannot set himself up in the analysand's mind as a substitute for God".[137] Freud rested his faith instead in science. Applying his science of psychoanalysis to religious conversion, he reduced it to secular terms in the case, for instance, of an American doctor who consulted him in the late 1920s. The experience had occurred, the doctor told Freud, after seeing a dead woman on a dissecting table. Initially he had reacted by doubting God's existence for, he argued, God could not possibly allow "this sweet-faced dear old woman" to suffer such a fate. But a few days later, the doctor wrote, "God made it clear to my soul that the Bible was His Word", and that Jesus was his "personal saviour".[138] Analyzing this in terms of his theory of the Oedipus complex, Freud interpreted the doctor's suddenly intensified religious faith as due to the sight of the old woman reviving his childhood longing for his mother and indignation against his father, against whom he said the doctor defended with his seemingly religious conversion experience of "submission to the will of God".[139]

Freud similarly reduced mysticism to secular defence. William James, as we have seen, argued that, in mystical states of mind, "we both become one with the Absolute and we become aware of our oneness".[140] Now, after Freud's rejection of religious experience as illusion, Rolland wrote insisting on the reality of the sense of oneness in mysticism as "the simple and direct fact of the feeling of the 'eternal' ". It has no "perceptible limits", he said, it is "oceanic".[141] Unlike

---

[134] Ibid. p. 54.

[135] Ibid. p. 56.

[136] See O. Pfister (1928/1993) The illusion of a future, *IJPA*, **74** pp. 557–79.

[137] To Pfister, 26 November 1927, in Meng and Freud pp. 117, 118.

[138] S. Freud (1928) A religious experience, **SE21** pp. 169–72, 169.

[139] Ibid. p. 171.

[140] W. James (1902) *The Varieties of Religious Experience*, London: Collins, 1960 p. 404.

[141] To Freud, 5 December 1927, in W. B. Parsons (1999) *The Enigma of the Oceanic Feeling: Revisioning the Psychoanalytic Theory of Mysticism*, New York: Oxford University Press, p. 36.

organized religion, he wrote, this experience was a major source of comfort and inspiration:

> All through my life, it has never failed me; and I have always found in it a source of vital renewal. In that sense, I can say that I am profoundly "religious" – without this constant state (like a sheet of water which I feel flushing under the bark) affecting in any way my critical faculties and my freedom to exercise them – even if that goes against the immediacy of the interior experience. In this way, without discomfort or contradiction, I can lead a "religious" life (in the sense of that prolonged feeling) and a life of critical reason (which is without illusion) . . . the sentiment I experience is imposed on me as a fact. It is a *contact*. And as I have recognized it to be identical (with multiple nuances) in a large number of living souls, it has helped me to understand that that was the true subterranean source of *religious energy* which, subsequently, has been collected, canalized and *dried up by the Churches*.[142]

Like William James and Romain Rolland, Freud too was critical of organized religion, just as, also like James, he was critical of organized medicine. He was determined to protect psychoanalysis from both. Hence the conjunction, he explained to Pfister, of his two essays, both published in 1927, defending non-medical "lay analysis" and criticizing religion as an "illusion". To this he added, apropos psychoanalysis, "I should like to hand it over to a profession which does not yet exist, a profession of *lay* curers of souls who need not be doctors and should not be priests".[143] But he was bothered by Rolland's objections to his dismissing mysticism as an illusion. "Your letter of December 5, 1927", he wrote, "containing your remarks about a feeling you describe as 'oceanic' has left me no peace".[144] He followed this with a letter thanking him for permission to quote him in a "new work" he was planning on the subject, adding "How remote from me are the worlds in which you move! To me mysticism is just as closed a book as music".[145]

Freud devoted the first chapter of his next book to mysticism. In it he located the origin of what Rolland called the oceanic experience in "primary narcissism", namely the baby's first loving oneness with his mother.[146] He argued that mystical experience derives from the baby at the breast not distinguishing "his ego from the external world as the source of sensations flowing in upon him".[147]

142 To Freud, 5 December 1927, in W. B. Parsons (1999) *The Enigma of the Oceanic Feeling: Revisioning the Psychoanalytic Theory of Mysticism*, New York: Oxford University Press, pp. 36–7.

143 To Pfister, 25 November 1928, in Meng and Freud p. 126.

144 To Rollan, 14 July 1929, in Freud 1961 p. 388.

145 Ibid. pp. 388, 389.

146 S. Freud (1914) On narcissism: An introduction, **SE**14 pp. 73–102, 88.

147 S. Freud (1930) *Civilization and its Discontents*, **SE**21 pp. 64–145, 66–7.

But however blissful this experience, its revival is risky. For Freud it threatened the fate described by Schiller in his poem, *The Diver*. The poem depicts a man diving into an "oceanic womb" that "boils and hisses . . . a gaping chasm . . . leading to the depths of hell". Freud accordingly ended his answer to Rolland by quoting the first two lines from the following stanza of Schiller's poem:

> Let him rejoice
> Who breathe up here in the roseate light!
> Far below all is fearful, of moment sad;
> Let no man tempt the immortals e'er try;
> Let him never desire the things to see
> That with terror and night they veil graciously.[148]

Freud remained wary of mysticism. In early 1930 he wrote to Rolland dismissing Jung as "a bit of a mystic", and also dismissing non-materially based intuition:

> Your mystics rely on it to teach them how to solve the riddle of the universe; we believe that it cannot reveal to us anything but primitive, instinctual impulses and attitudes – highly valuable for an embriology of the soul when correctly interpreted, but worthless for orientation in the alien, external world.[149]

Subsequently he was arguably more sympathetic to mysticism. He likened the occultism of spiritualism, telepathy, and thought-transference to psychoanalysis in so far as they too seek to make conscious the unconscious of another. He also likened mysticism to psychoanalysis in so far as both seek to free the truth of the id and ego from the superego. Or, as he put it,

> It is easy to imagine, too, that certain mystical practices may succeed in upsetting the normal relations between the different regions of the mind, so that, for instance, perception may be able to grasp happenings in the depths of the ego and in the id which were otherwise inaccessible to it. . . . the therapeutic efforts of psychoanalysis have chosen a similar line of approach. Its intention is, indeed, to strengthen the ego, to make it more independent of the super-ego, to widen its field of perception and enlarge its organization, so that it can appropriate fresh portions of the id. Where id was, there ego shall be.[150]

Or, in German, "*Wo Es war, soll Ich werden*" – "Where it was I shall become".

More often, however, Freud continued to dismiss mysticism, as he had long dismissed religion, as a defence. He told Romain Rolland, for instance, of a seeming mystical experience occurring to him on first seeing the Acropolis

---

[148] In Parsons p. 46.

[149] To Rolland, 19 January 1930, in Freud 1961 pp. 392–3.

[150] S. Freud (1933) *New Introductory Lectures on Psycho-Analysis*, **SE22** pp. 5–182, 79–80.

with his younger brother, Alexander, in 1904. He described the experience as one of incredulity: "So all this really *does* exist, just as we learnt at school!" It was like reacting to seeing the Loch Ness monster, Freud said, with "So it really *does* exist – the sea-serpent we've never believed in!" It was the experience, he said, of something "too good to be true".[151] It was indeed too good to be true. It was false, said Freud. It was an illusion conjured up as defence against his anxiety about surpassing his father who, having had no secondary education, would have known little of the wonders of ancient Greece.

The same year, 1936, as Freud wrote to Rolland of his quasi-mystical experience on the Acropolis, Freud's daughter, Anna, who had become a psychoanalyst, gave him, for his eightieth birthday, a book by her about psychoanalysis.[152] In it she altered psychoanalysis into a method of therapy aimed at revising and firming up the defences of the ego and superego against instincts of love and sex in the id. Freud now adopted her version of psychoanalysis. If, like education and government, psychoanalysis was not to become an "impossible" profession, he said, the defences of the patient should be firmed up. So too should those of the analyst, if necessary through the analyst having further analysis to deal with the instinctual demands unleashed by "preoccupation with all the repressed material which struggles for freedom".[153]

Freud's essay to this effect was published in June 1937. The same year two of the three essays constituting his last book about religion, *Moses and Monotheism*, were published. As in Freud's first book about religion, Freud bent historical truth in these essays to his psychoanalytic presuppositions. Against the evidence, he argued that Moses was an Egyptian who had served as a district governor to Akhenaton, the pharaoh who introduced monotheism into Egypt. When Akhenaton died and his monotheistic religion was crushed, Moses took the Jewish people he governed out of Egypt. But he too was overthrown. He was murdered, Freud speculated. The truth of his murder, Freud went on, is only not known because it has been defensively repressed. But it is evident, Freud claimed, from the readiness of Jews to accept blame for Christ's crucifixion, and from their obedience to Moses's commandment not to make graven images of God.[154] Matter thereby became spirit. God became breath,

---

[151] S. Freud (1936) A disturbance of memory on the Acropolis, **SE22** pp. 239–48, 241, 242.

[152] A. Freud (1936) *The Ego and Mechanisms of Defence*, London: Hogarth, 1968.

[153] S. Freud (1937) Analysis terminable and interminable, **SE23** pp. 216–53, 248, 249.

[154] "Thou shalt not make unto thee any graven image, or any likeness *of any thing* that *is* in heaven above, or that *is* in the earth beneath, or that *is* in the water under the earth: Thou shalt not bow down theyself to them, nor serve them" – *Exodus* ch. 20 verses 4–5 – emphasis in original.

"invisible like a gale of wind or like the soul". This heralded, he said, the victory of paternal over maternal descent established through abstract reason – through "memories, reflections and inferences" – rather than through the sensuous bodily reality in terms of which mothers know to whom they have given birth.[155] Freud however concluded with his now convinced belief in adapting the ego's defences against the id. He warned against religious experience giving the id shape. He compared the pious believer's overwhelming feelings of something hidden being revealed in his experience of God to the wishes repressed by children into the unconscious. "[O]nly religious ecstasy", he said, can bring it back.[156]

He initially resisted publication of these essays in book form lest, with the rise of fascism in Italy and Germany, it might lose the protection of psychoanalysis in Austria by offending its Catholic church with his conclusion reducing, as he put it, "religion to a neurosis".[157] Appeasing his fellow-countrymen, however, soon became irrelevant. On 12 March 1938 Hitler's troops invaded Austria. Freud was persuaded to leave, via Paris, for London where, that June, he wrote that he now felt free to have his *Moses and Monotheism* essays published. In early August his daughter, Anna, presented some of their material to that year's international congress of psychoanalysis in Paris. The same month he noted, "Mysticism is the obscure self-perception of the realm outside the ego, of the id".[158] Allying mysticism with the nothingness sought by the death instinct, he described it, as seeking "a reduction, at bottom the extinction perhaps, of the tensions of instinctual needs (that is *Nirvana*)".[159]

But the book was not published in Freud's lifetime. He had been suffering with cancer since 1923. Just before midnight on 23 September 1939, which happened that year to fall on the holiest day of the Jewish calendar, Yom Kippur, the Day of Atonement, Freud died. At his funeral three days later Ernest Jones concluded, "And so we take leave of a man whose like we shall not know again. From our hearts we thank him for having lived; for having done; and for having loved".[160]

Inspired by love of Fliess and others, I have argued, Freud discovered means of treating the ills done by the defences against sex and love of neurosis,

---

155 S. Freud (1939) *Moses and Monotheism*, **SE23** pp. 7–137, 117–8.

156 Ibid. p. 134.

157 Ibid. p. 55.

158 Dated 22 August 1938, **SE23** p. 300.

159 S. Freud (1940) *An Outline of Psycho-Analysis*, **SE23** pp. 144–207, 198.

160 E. Jones (1957) *Sigmund Freud: Life and Work, Vol. III*, London: Hogarth, p. 265.

psychosis, and organized religion through addressing the "transference-love" awakened in patients by analysis. Disappointment in, and loss of those he loved, I have also argued, perhaps contributed to his subsequently dismissing as an illusion the oneness with another of being in love, and the oceanic oneness with the otherness of God or the universe of religious and mystical experience. Betraying his initial insights regarding the importance of psychoanalysis freeing sex and love from secular and religious repression, Freud focused in his final work on psychoanalysis as a means of shoring up the repression exercised by the defences of the ego and superego. Nevertheless – as Pfister, Jones, and many others have noted – Freud did much for love. So too did Jung, whose development of the conjunction of psychoanalysis with religion I will detail next.

Chapter 3

Carl Jung

Transforming libido

Just as William James emphasized the transforming therapeutic effects of religious experience, so too did Jung. Whereas Freud was pessimistic about the healing effects of therapy – anticipating that, at best, it might convert "hysterical misery into common unhappiness"[1] – Jung was much more optimistic. He wrote of transforming the libido through visual and symbolic imagery. He also wrote of the transforming effect of religious experience reconnecting us with what he called the "archetypes" of God and the "soul-image" (anima in men, animus in women) in "the collective unconscious". Furthermore he emphasized the healing effect of the mutual influence of patients and therapists on each other. In doing so, I will argue, he was particularly inspired by his love of one of his patients, Sabina Spielrein.

Paradoxically, however, Jung also lost sight of the intersubjective, I/Thou, character of religious experience in reducing God and the soul to unchanging, thing-like figures in the collective unconscious. He argued, in effect, that these figures are true for all time, unlike Freud who, through free association, sought to enable patients to become conscious of figures and fantasies in their unconscious so they could test their truth against consciously perceived reality. Jung too was scientifically-minded. But he tended to subordinate science to spirituality and to religion, and it is with this that I will begin.

Religious beginnings

Jung's paternal grandfather, also called Carl Gustav Jung, was a doctor and as rector of Basel University, sought, unsuccessfully, to found a chair of psychiatry there. Many of Jung's other forebears, including his father, Paul, were parsons in the Swiss reformed church. Jung's maternal grandfather, Samuel Preiswerk, was Bishop of Basel. He had visions, and some of his children were credited with being in touch with spirits and with having second sight.

---

[1] S. Freud (1895) *Studies on Hysteria*, SE2 p. 305.

Jung himself was born in Kesswil on Lake Constance on 26 July 1875. He too had visions. He was an isolated, only child, until the birth of his sister, Gertrud, when he was 9. Earlier, his mother had been hospitalized with depression in Basel, when the family moved near there when Jung was 3. He later remembered from this time sharing a room with his father and seeing "frightening influences" coming from his mother's room in the form of "a faintly luminous, indefinite figure whose head detached itself from the neck and floated along in front of it, in the air, like a little moon".[2] He also recalled himself as a child, cradled in his father's arms, having a vision in which, he said, he saw "a glowing blue circle about the size of the full moon, and inside it moved golden figures which I thought were angels".[3]

Other memories included comforting himself by carving a mannequin out of the end of ruler, colouring and dressing it, putting it in a pencil-case for its bed, and hiding it secretly, together with a stone – "*his* stone" – in the attic of his childhood home.[4] Thinking of it, visiting it, consoled him, he said, "whenever I had done something wrong or my feelings had been hurt, or when my father's irritability or my mother's invalidism oppressed me".[5]

Staying with friends of the family in early adolescence, he experienced himself as what William James might have called a "divided self". He felt divided between what he called "two different persons" – a schoolboy and an eighteenth-century, old-man version of himself.[6] This was followed by what James might have called a religious conversion experience. Coming out of secondary school into the bright noon-day sun, and seeing the glittering roof of Basel Cathedral, he thought "The word is beautiful and the church is beautiful, and God made all this and sits above it far away in the blue sky on a golden throne and . . .".[7] At first he felt too terrified to go on. And then, thinking he must trust to God's will, he dared pursue his vision, whereupon he saw God sitting on a golden throne, "high above the world and from under the throne an enormous turd falls upon the sparkling new roof, shatters it, and breaks the walls of the cathedral asunder".[8]

---

[2] C. G. Jung (1961) *Memories, Dreams, Reflections*, London: Fontana, 1967 p. 33.

[3] Ibid. p. 34.

[4] Ibid. p. 36.

[5] Ibid. p. 37.

[6] Ibid. p. 50.

[7] Ibid. p. 52.

[8] Ibid. p. 56.

Just as William James felt that, unlike his father, he dared countenance evil as well as good, so did Jung. Unlike James, however, Jung experienced God. He now knew after his vision, he said, that "God could do stupendous things to me, things of fire and unearthly light".[9] He now understood, as he put it, that God was "one of the most certain and immediate of experiences".[10] It was as if "a breath of the great world of stars and endless space . . . a spirit had invisibly entered . . . with the halo of a *numen*".[11] He described this *numen* as the background of his "No. 2" personality. He also dreaded being overwhelmed by this second self. In a dream he pictured it as "a gigantic black figure" following him, threatening to put out "a tiny light" cupped in the hand of his "No. 1" self.[12] To keep it alight, he decided he must study science. But because of his family's poverty and his consequent need to earn a living, he opted instead for medicine.

On 18 April 1895 he registered as a medical student at Basel University. The same June he also started doing spiritualist experiments at home with his thirteen-and-a-half-year-old cousin, Helene (Helly) Preiswerk – experiments that were interrupted by Jung's father, Paul, becoming ill. Previously Paul had suffered with depression for which he had sought psychiatric treatment. Now he became physically ill and on 18 January 1896, he died. Later that year Jung's spiritualist experiments with Helly were resumed. Inspired, it seems by love of Jung, Helly talked in her trances in the voice of their shared grandfather, Samuel Preiswerk, and in the voice of a sister of the seventeenth century Swedish mystic, Swedenborg, whose work, like William James' father, Jung very much admired. Speaking about Swedenborg's "clairvoyant vision" of the great fire of 1756 in Stockholm to a student society in May 1897, Jung emphasized the importance of scientifically investigating the spiritual as well as the material world.[13]

Jung's enthusiasm for spiritual and psychical research contributed to his becoming interested in psychiatry. Reading Krafft-Ebing's textbook on the subject convinced him, he said, that psychiatry proved the reality of "the collision of nature and spirit".[14] After passing his final examination at Basel University on 26 November 1900, he got a job in psychiatry at the Burghölzli mental hospital in Zurich, and started work there on 10 December 1900.

....

[9] Ibid. p. 72.

[10] Ibid. p. 80.

[11] Ibid. p. 84.

[12] Ibid. p. 108.

[13] C. G. Jung (1897) Some thoughts on psychology, **CWA** pp. 21–47.

[14] Jung 1961 p. 130.

Inspiring Freud

Jung now learnt about Freud. At the request of the Burghölzli's director, Eugen Bleuler, he presented a summary, on 25 January 1901, of Freud's account of dreams.[15] Bleuler also supervised Jung's dissertation recounting his spiritualist experiments with Helly.[16] Writing up his findings, Jung drew on Freud's theory of the unconscious. He also drew, as did James in his 1901–1902 lectures on religious experience, on the findings of Pierre Janet, Theodore Flournoy and others. Bringing their discoveries together with those of Freud, Jung argued that his cousin Helly's spirits resulted from repressed emotionally charged ideas erupting as hallucinated independent personalities.

He defended his dissertation in April 1902, qualified as a doctor that July, and then went to Paris where he attended Janet's lectures at the Salpêtrière. The next year, on 14 February 1903, he married Emma Rauschenburg, the daughter of a rich industrialist, with whom he had five children.[17] Meanwhile Bleuler's enthusiasm for Freud's work gave Freud reason to write to Fliess again. He wrote asking him to contribute to a scientific journal he was planning. The time was now ripe, he said, given increasing agreement with his views, evident from "an absolutely stunning recognition of my point of view in a book review . . . by an official psychiatrist, Bleuler, in Zurich".[18]

Bleuler meantime had been encouraging Jung, together with a colleague, Franz Riklin, in conducting word association tests in which they measured the reaction times of patients in producing words in association to words presented to them in the tests. They thereby sought to root psychical reality in measurable "feeling-toned complexes".[19] Jung also used these tests, together with Freud's free association method, to diagnose and treat what Jung believed to be the repressed or fragmented eruptions of these complexes in patients with hysteria and schizophrenia. He included examples in two books – *Diagnostic Association Studies* and *The Psychology of Dementia Praecox* – which he sent to Freud.

---

[15] C. G. Jung (1901) Sigmund Freud: "On Dreams", **CW18** pp. 361–68.

[16] C. G. Jung (1902) On the psychology and pathology of so-called occult phenomena, **CW1** pp. 1–88.

[17] Agathe born on 16 December 1904, Gret born on 1 June 1906, Franz born on 1 December 1908, Marianne born on 17 September 1910, and Helene born on 14 March 1914.

[18] To Fliess, 26 April 1904, in J. M. Masson (1985) *The Complete Letters of Sigmund Freud to Wilhelm Fliess 1887–1904*, Cambridge: Harvard University Press, p. 461.

[19] C. G. Jung and F. Riklin (1906) *Diagnostic Association Studies*, **CW2** pp. 1–271, 188–317.

Freud was delighted. He told Jung that his book about *dementia praecox* (the term coined by Kraepelin for a condition later called schizophrenia by Bleuler) was "the richest and most significant contribution to my labours that has ever come to my attention".[20] Soon after the two men met for the first time in Vienna, in early March 1907, when Jung attended a meeting of the Vienna Psycho-Analytical Society at which Freud first presented his theory linking obsessional neurosis with religion (see p. 46 above).[21] The next day Freud and Jung talked long into the night. Soon they wrote to each other with increasing frequency.

That September they met again, this time at the first International Congress of Psychiatry and Neurology in Amsterdam. Here Jung presented, without mentioning her name, the case of Sabina Spielrein. He recounted her treatment in terms of Freud's theories about dreams and infantile sexuality, and argued that her symptoms were rooted in anal fantasies from infancy.[22] In a subsequent letter to Freud he told him about his own sexual experiences as a child. "Dear Professor Freud," he wrote,

> my veneration of you has something of the character of a "religious" crush. Though it does not really bother me, I still feel it is disgusting and ridiculous because of its undeniable erotic undertones. This abominable feeling comes from the fact that as a boy I was the victim of a sexual assault by a man I once worshipped.[23]

Shortly after this a couple of essays by Freud on similar topics – homosexuality and anal eroticism – to those described by Jung in this letter and in his Amsterdam paper were published.[24]

This was followed by Jung and Freud meeting again, this time at the first congress of the International Psychoanalytic Association (IPA) held in Salzburg. Here it was decided to establish the IPA's own journal, of which Jung became the first editor. Here too Freud presented his Rat Man case, and Jung spoke about dementia praecox. Soon after this one of the psychiatrist Emil Kraepelin's colleagues in Munich, Otto Gross, who had attended the Salzburg conference, went mad. He was hospitalized in the Burghölzli where Jung became intensely involved with him. He called him his "twin brother".[25] But no sooner had he seemingly begun to cure him than Gross ran away.

---

20 To Jung, 1 January 1907, in W. McGuire (1974) *The Freud/Jung Letters*, London: Hogarth, p. 17.

21 S. Freud (1907) Obsessive actions and religious practices, **SE9** pp. 117–27.

22 C. G. Jung (1908) The Freudian theory of hysteria, **CW4** pp. 10–24.

23 To Freud, 28 October 1907, in McGuire pp. 94, 95.

24 S. Freud (1908) Hysterical phantasies and their relation to bisexuality, **SE9**, pp. 157–66; S. Freud (1908) Character and anal erotism, **SE9** pp. 169–75.

25 J. Kerr (1994) *A Most Dangerous Method*, London: Sinclair-Stevenson, p. 187.

Upset by this, Jung became increasingly involved with Freud, whom he invited to stay with him that September while his wife and children were away. Pleased at the prospect, Freud wrote, "My selfish purpose is to persuade you to continue and complete my work by applying to psychoses what I have begun with neuroses".[26] Jung duly obliged by introducing Freud to his patients, including one, Babette, whose case Jung had detailed in his 1906 book about applying Freud's theory and method in understanding and treating psychotic patients.

Jung continued to use Freud's ideas in his psychiatric work. Freud, however, was not entirely happy with Jung's word association method, telling Pfister, "I make practically no use of the association technique, and see no advantage in it over my own technique of free association".[27] Pfister's own work, he wrote, strengthened his "impression that the suggested association technique [of Jung], though indispensable in cases of *dementia praecox*, has no special value in the analysis of neurotics, and is in no way preferable to free association".[28]

Meanwhile the first issue of the IPA's journal had appeared, including an article by Jung rooting religious ideas in early childhood complexes about the father:

> These [father complexes] are the roots of the first religious sublimations. In the place of the father with his constellating virtues and faults there appears on the one hand an altogether sublime deity, and on the other hand the devil.[29]

A similar father complex seemed to haunt Freud's relation with Jung. On 20 August 1909 they met in Bremen, where ancient skeletons had recently been discovered. Jung talked about the discovery, at which Freud seemed upset. Nevertheless Jung continued talking about the skeletons whereupon Freud fainted, an occurrence he later attributed to his experiencing Jung's talk as expressing a death wish against him as Jung's ersatz father.

From Bremen they went with Ferenczi to give lectures in Clark University in Massachusetts. In his lectures Freud adopted Jung's terminology. Speaking about the sexual feelings of parents for their children, and about children's sexual wish to replace one parent with the other, Freud called this constellation of feelings and its repression the "nuclear complex" of every neurosis.[30]

---

26 To Jung, 13 August 1908, in McGuire p. 168.

27 To Pfister, 18 March 1909, in H. Meng and E. Freud (1963) *Psycho-Analysis and Faith*, London: Hogarth, p. 17.

28 To Pfister, 18 March 1909, ibid. p. 22.

29 C. G. Jung (1909) The significance of the father in the destiny of the individual, **CW4** pp. 301–23, 321 n. 22.

30 S. Freud (1910) *Five Lectures on Psycho-Analysis*, **SE11** pp. 9–55, 47.

The two men also analysed each other's dreams, including one of Jung's in which he pictured himself descending from an upper storey of a house to a medieval ground floor, and then on through a Roman cellar into a prehistoric cave littered with bones, broken pottery, and two ancient disintegrating skulls. Freud, it seems, interpreted the skulls, as he had Jung's talk about the Bremen skeletons, as expressing Jung's death wishes against him. Jung himself, however, said the dream expressed and revived his already existing enthusiasm for archaeology.

Freud too was interested in archaeology and likened it to psychoanalysis in his account of the Rat Man case published in the IPA's journal that summer.[31] On their return from the USA both he and Jung became increasingly interested in both archaeology and in mythology and symbolism. Freud now added a section about symbolism in a new edition of *The Interpretation of Dreams* which was published that year. But he also warned "against over-estimating the importance of symbols in dream-interpretation". He warned "against restricting the work of translating dreams merely to translating symbols and against abandoning the technique of use of the dreamer's associations".[32] Jung, however, moved towards increasingly emphasizing symbolism. He told Freud he was "immersed" in reading its history, about "the Mother–Mary cult", and so on.[33] He planned to root in mythology "the nuclear complex of neurosis",[34] a notion Freud took up in terms of "the castration complex in myth".[35] To this Jung replied anticipating his later theory of the collective unconscious. "What we now find in the individual psyche – in compressed, stunted, or one-sidedly differentiated form", he envisaged, "may be seen spread out in all its fullness in times past".[36]

These developments in both men's thinking were reflected in Freud's account of unconscious symbolism in the art and life of Leonardo da Vinci.[37] He also adopted Jung's terminology in an essay in which he introduced the term "Oedipus complex" for the first time.[38] Meanwhile Jung began formulating a theory about two forms of thinking – verbal and symbolic (subsequently rooted neurologically by Jungians in the brain's dominant and non-dominant

---

[31] S. Freud (1909) Notes upon a case of obsessional neurosis, **SE10** pp. 155–249.

[32] S. Freud (1909) in *Interpretation of Dreams*, **SE5** pp. 359–60.

[33] To Freud, 8 November 1909, in McGuire p. 258.

[34] To Freud, 15 November 1909, ibid. p. 263.

[35] To Jung, 21 November 1909, ibid. p. 265.

[36] To Freud, 2 December 1909, ibid. p. 269.

[37] S. Freud (1910) *Leonardo da Vinci and a Memory of his Childhood*, **SE11** pp. 59–137.

[38] S. Freud (1910) A special type of choice of object made by men, **SE11** pp. 165–75.

hemispheres).[39] In January 1910 he gave a lecture in which he described verbal thinking as "logical" and outward-directed, and symbolic thinking as "emotionally toned, pictorial and wordless . . . inner-directed rumination on materials belonging to the past archaic, unconscious".[40]

Jung developed this theory further at a meeting of Swiss psychiatrists in Herisau on 16 May 1910. In his lecture he spoke of dreams returning us from verbal to symbolic thinking. He told Freud of the "great applause" greeting his Herisau lecture.[41] It prompted Freud, it seems, to reiterate his rather different theory of pleasure- and reality-based thinking which he had first been inspired to draft following his September 1895 meeting with Fliess. In his resulting essay, Freud argued that art seeks to reconcile reality and pleasure whilst religion offers consolation for repressing pleasure with the promise of heaven when we die.[42]

Meeting with Jung in Munich, on 26 December 1910, Freud also urged him never to abandon his sexual theory. It must be retained, he said, as "an unshaekable bulwark . . . [a]gainst the black tide of mud . . . occultism".[43] Perhaps Freud was particularly concerned to emphasize this because Jung was increasingly dissenting from his sexual theory in work he was now doing for a book, later published as *Transformations and Symbols of the Libido*. This brings me to Sabina Spielrein.

Sabina Spielrein

Sabina Spielrein was the oldest child and only daughter of a wealthy Jewish businessman. Born in Rostov-on-Don, in Russia, in 1885, Sabina, it seems from Jung's account of her case, was early preoccupied with anal fantasies. By middle childhood, it seems, she also became so immersed in masturbating and erotic fantasies of being beaten by her father that she could not bear to look at anyone. In her teens she also suffered terrible fits of weeping, laughing, and screaming, alternating with bouts of depression, for which her mother took her for treatment to Zurich. Here, on 17 August 1904, Sabina was transferred from a private psychiatric clinic to the Burghölzli.

[39] E. Christopher (2002) Whose unconscious is it, anyway? *Journal of the British Association of Psychotherapists*, **40** pp. 131–44.

[40] To Freud, 1 March 1910, in McGuire pp. 298, 299.

[41] To Freud, 24 May 1910, ibid. p. 319.

[42] S. Freud (1911) Formulations on the two principles of mental functioning, **SE12** pp. 218–26.

[43] Jung 1961 p. 173.

Jung's analysis of Sabina at the Burghölzli was evidently successful. By April 1905 she was well enough to register as a medical student at Zurich University, and following her discharge from the Burghölzli (at the beginning of June) moved into a boarding house from where she started attending classes. The same year Jung became a lecturer at the university, and gave his inaugural lecture there that October. He and Speilrein now became close friends. She was evidently also inspired by him. Writing in the third person to him the next summer, she said of his lecture and psychoanalysis:

> There you were, able to create so much enthusiasm and feeling . . . you treated the patients with so much care and love I was completely transformed, soft and warm towards people. . . . [your letters] stimulate the better part of her personality so that at a moment of weakness I can think of you and become stronger.[44]

She wrote to her mother of the healing effect of loving him:

> I am now somewhat tired but completely at peace. I am deliriously happy as never before in my life . . . You have probably guessed that the cause of all this is Junga. I visited him today.[45]

Perhaps Jung had something of this in mind when he wrote of the value of introducing a new complex in therapy to free the patient from "the complex of the illness".[46] He included the essay in which this conclusion appeared, together with one of his earliest letters to Freud in which he also dwelt at length on Spielrein's case:

> At the risk of boring you, I must abreact my most recent experience. I am currently treating an hysteric with your method. Difficult case, a 20-year-old Russian girl student, ill for 6 years. First trauma between the 3rd and 4th year. Saw her father spanking her older brother on the bare bottom. Powerful impression. Couldn't help thinking afterwards that she had defecated on her father's hand. From the 4th–7th year convulsive attempts to defecate on her own feet, in the following manner: she sat on the floor with one foot beneath her, pressed her heel against her anus and tried to defecate and at the same time to prevent defecation. Often retained the stool for 2 weeks in this way! Has no idea how she hit upon this peculiar business; says it was completely instinctive, and accompanied by blissfully shuddersome feelings. Later this phenomenon was superseded by vigorous masturbation. I should be extremely grateful if you would tell me in a few words what you think of this story.[47]

---

[44] To Jung, 1906, in Z. Lothane (1999) Tender love and transference: Unpublished letters of C. G. Jung and Sabina Spielrein, *IJPA*, **80** pp. 1189–1204, 1193, 1194.

[45] To her mother, 26 August 1905, ibid. p. 1191.

[46] C. G. Jung (1906) Association, dream, and hysterical symptom, **CW2** pp. 353–407, 407.

[47] To Freud, 23 October 1906, in McGuire p. 7.

Freud immediately replied by interpreting the case as one of "anal auto-erotism" and "infantile fixation of the libido on the father".[48] A "decisive change", however, now occurred in Spielrein's analysis.[49] Her anal fantasies – or complex – became transformed into a figure which recurred in her dreams, and which she associated with the hero, Siegfried, of Wagner's opera, *The Ring*. Writing later to Freud about what she then referred to as her "Siegfried complex", she said:

> When I confessed this complex to Dr. Jung for the first time, he treated me with tender-est friendship, like a father, if you will. He admitted to me that from time to time he, too, had to consider such matters in connection with me (i.e., his affinity with me and the possible consequences), that such wishes are not alien to him . . . the thought of his great love made me want to keep him perfectly "pure".[50]

Soon Spielrein came to understand psychoanalysis, at least its treatment of neurosis, as a matter of transforming the neurotic's complexes just as Jung had written in the essay which he had included with his letter to Freud about her case. In an unpublished essay in her diary, "On love, death, and transforma-tion",[51] the first two parts of which seem to have been written in the summer of 1907, she argued that mental life is governed by two fundamental tendencies: the power of persisting complexes, and "the instinct for transformation".[52] She went on to argue that, in seeking to objectify and master our complexes, we seek to find similar complexes in others. Sharing complexes with them evokes feelings of sympathy, similarity, and sexual attraction. But, she went on, since sex, unlike love, operates universally – at the level of the species – it is contrary to, and destructive of our individuality. Nevertheless, she claimed, its destruct-iveness can be circumvented by sacrificing oneself for a cause. This self-sacrifice, she said, is inspired by an instinct for transformation. She added that this instinct also expresses itself in love, intimacy, and art.[53] Addressing herself to Jung in her "transformation" essay, she wrote:

> Art is only a complex which has found its independence or which "having turned wild, wants to express itself fully" (your words) – or "wants to be transformed" (my words).[54]

---

[48] To Jung, 17 October 1906, ibid. p. 8.

[49] J. Kerr p. 161.

[50] To Freud, 1909, in A. Carotenuto (1984) *A Secret Symmetry*, London: Routledge, p. 108.

[51] S. Spielrein (1906/7) Unedited extracts from a diary, *Journal of Analytical Psychology*, 2001, 46, pp. 155–71.

[52] Kerr p. 166.

[53] Ibid. p. 167.

[54] Spielrein 1906/7 p. 159.

The same summer Jung wrote to Freud about Sabina's use of art in therapy. Without using her name, he described a poem she said kept going round in her mind:

> The poem is about a prisoner whose sole companion is a bird in a cage. The prisoner is animated only by one wish: sometime in his life, as his noblest deed, to give some creature its freedom. He opens the cage and lets his beloved bird fly out. What is the patient's greatest wish? "Once in my life I would like to help someone to perfect freedom through psychoanalytical treatment". In her dreams she is condensed with me. She admits that actually her greatest wish is to have a child by me.[55]

By the next summer, 1908, Jung had become increasingly involved with Sabina. He wrote, for instance, "you have vigorously taken my unconscious into your hands with your saucy letters", and suggested a time they meet to "find a clear way out from the turmoil we are in".[56] In another letter he wrote, "You cannot imagine how much it means to me to have hopes of loving a person whom I must not condemn, and who does not condemn herself, to being smothered in the banality of habit".[57] That summer Spielrein went on holiday to Russia to where Jung wrote to her, relieved she had written:

> Your letter made me happy and calm . . . As per your letter, everything is good and lovely; I delight in your happiness . . . My own mood sings like a volcano, now everything looks golden, now it looks grey. Your letter was like a ray of sun through the clouds.[58]

In October Spielrein returned to Zurich, where, at the beginning of December, Jung's long-wanted son was born. Three days later he wrote to Spielrein, apologizing for having mistreated her professionally, begging her not to take revenge, and imploring her to meet with him, adding:

> I am looking for a person who can love without punishing, imprisoning and draining the other person; I am seeking this as yet unrealized type who will manage to separate love from social advantage or disadvantage, so that love may always be an end unto itself, not just a means for achieving another end. . . . It is my misfortune that my life means nothing to me without the joy of love, of tempestuous, eternally changing love . . . . Return to me, in this moment of my need, some of the love and guilt and altruism which I was able to give you at the time of your illness. Now it is I who am ill.[59]

Writing to her mother at this time, Spielrein said

> he has fallen in love with me . . . Twice in a row he became so emotional in my presence that tears just rolled down his face! . . . Then he starts reproaching himself

---

55 To Freud, 6 July 1907, in McGuire p. 72.

56 To Spielrein, 20 June 1908, in Kerr p. 196.

57 To Spielrein, 30 June 1908, ibid. p. 197.

58 To Spielrein, 12 August 1908, in Lothane p. 1194.

59 To Spielrein, 4 December 1908, in Kerr p. 205.

endlessly for his feelings, for example, that I am something sacred for him, that he is ready to beg forgiveness, etc . . . Then I get a post card and a letter in one day, that I should not be sad, and last Friday he came again. Poetry again, and as usual, will I ever in my life forgive him what he had concocted with me . . . The question for me is whether to surrender with all my being to this violent vortex of life and to be happy while the sun is shining, or, when the gloom descends, to let the feeling become transferred to a child and science.[60]

But then, early the next year, everything changed. In mid-January 1909 Spielrein's mother received an anonymous letter (probably from Jung's wife) warning her to save her daughter from Jung. She wrote to Jung, who in turn wrote to Bleuler tendering his resignation from the Burghölzli. He also replied to Spielrein's mother acknowledging that when his professional relationship with her daughter had ended they had become friends and, as often happens in such cases, he said, "something more" had entered into their relationship.[61]

He also evidently told Sabina that they could no longer meet in her room in town. Their meetings would have to be confined to appointments in his office. She missed the next three. And when, at her fourth appointment, on 26 February 1909, he told her he had been too good to her, that she wanted too much, and that they must analyse why this was so, she attacked him, drew blood, and ran away. Frightened at what she might do next, Jung replied to Freud's telegram announcing the publication of the first issue of the IPA journal explaining that he had not written sooner because he was preoccupied with one of his patients having "kicked up a vile scandal solely because I denied myself the pleasure of giving her a child".[62] The same day he quit the Burghölzli, and at the end of May moved into a new house built for his family in a rural part of a village, Küsnach (later spelt Küsnacht) by Lake Zurich.

Five days later Spielrein wrote to Freud asking to meet him. Freud accordingly asked Jung who she was, at which Jung explained that she was the "test case" he had written to him about in October 1906 and described in his talk in Amsterdam in September 1907. She was now taking revenge on him, he said, by spreading a rumour that he was getting divorced and marrying a student. Her case and that of Otto Gross, he said, were "bitter experiences. To none of my patients have I extended so much friendship and from none have I reaped so much sorrow".[63]

---

[60] To her mother, end of 1908, ibid. pp. 1196–7.

[61] Reported by Spielrein to Freud, 11 June 1909, in Carotenuto p. 94.

[62] To Freud, 7 March 1909, in McGuire p. 207.

[63] To Freud, 4 June 1909, ibid. p. 229.

Freud made light of the affair. He told Jung he too had had similar experiences. They did no lasting damage. Indeed quite the reverse. "They help us", he said, "to develop the thick skin we need and to dominate 'counter-transference', which is after all a permanent problem for us; they teach us to displace our own affects to best advantage".[64] This was followed by Freud's first published account of counter-transference, in which he warned analysts to guard against it through continuing self-analysis.[65] A couple of years later he added a further warning:

> I cannot advise my colleagues too urgently to model themselves during psycho-analytic treatment on the surgeon, who puts aside all feeling, even his human sympathy, and concentrates his mental forces on the single aim of performing the operation as skilfully as possible. . . . The justification for requiring this emotional coldness in the analyst is that it creates the most advantageous conditions for both parties: for the doctor a desirable protection for his own emotional life and for the patient the largest amount of help that we can give him to-day. A surgeon of earlier times took as his motto the words: "*Je le pansai, Dieu le guérit*". [I dressed his wounds, God cured him.] The analyst should be content with something similar.[66]

Freud might urge analysts to be emotionally cold towards their patients, and he also evidently initially made light of the damage done to Spielrein by Jung. Spielrein was less calm. The same day Jung's family joined him in their new home in Küsnach she wrote to Freud in a letter which she never sent:

> When one thinks that this same person once wrote to me, "Your letter came like a ray of sun amid the clouds", . . . or "How happy I am to know a person with a magnificent spirit", etc., that he gave me his diary to read . . . that only a short time ago we could sit in speechless ecstasy for hours . . . My love for him transcended our affinity, until he could stand it no longer and wanted "poetry". For many reasons I could not and did not want to resist. But when he asked me how I pictured what would happen next (because of the "consequences"), I said that first love has no desires, that I had nothing in mind and did not want to go beyond a kiss, which I could also do without, if need be.[67]

A week later she met with Jung, who then wrote to Freud of the wrong he had done her in thinking she had been spreading rumours about him.

> The day before yesterday she turned up at my house and had a very decent talk with me, during which it transpired that the rumour buzzing about me does not emanate from her at all. . . . Caught in my delusion that I was the victim of the sexual wiles of

---

64 To Jung, 7 June 1909, ibid. p. 231.

65 S. Freud (1910) The future prospects of psycho-analytic therapy, **SE11** pp. 141–51, 145.

66 S. Freud (1912) Recommendations to physicians practising psycho-analysis, **SE12** pp. 11–120, 115.

67 To Freud, 12 June 1909, in Carotenuto p. 96.

my patient . . . [and] in view of the fact that the patient had shortly before been my friend and enjoyed my full confidence, my action was a piece of knavery which I very reluctantly confess to you as my father.[68]

He asked Freud to forgive him for dragging him into this "imbroglio". Whether or not Freud forgave him, Spielrein evidently did. They continued to be friends. But she was wary of becoming sexually involved with him, mindful perhaps, as she wrote in her diary, of her mother's observation that "it is impossible for my friend [Jung] and me to remain friends once we have given each other our love".[69] She wrote of their meeting:

> The most important outcome of our discussion was that we both loved each other fervently again. My friend said we would always have to be careful not to fall in love again; we would always be dangerous to each other. He admitted to me that so far he knew no female who could replace me. It was as if he had a necklace in which all his other admirers were – pearls, and I – the medallion. . . . Then he became more and more intense. At the end he pressed my hands to his heart several times and said this should mark the beginning of a new era.[70]

By the next autumn she was preoccupied not only with Jung but also with her dissertation, and with Bleuler's seeming neglect of her as her dissertation supervisor. She was relieved when Bleuler suggested she send her dissertation to Jung in the hope that he might publish it in the IPA journal.[71] She wrote of her willingness "to die for him [Jung], to sacrifice my honour for him . . . [and of] the child I wanted to give him".[72] They discussed her dissertation. In it, just as Jung had discussed two forms of thinking (verbal and symbolic) in his May 1910 Herisau lecture, she too discussed two forms of thinking. In her diary she noted his reaction to such similarities between them:

> He was deeply stirred by the parallels in our thinking and feeling. He told me that seeing this worries him, because that is how I make him fall in love with him . . . he did not want to love me. Now he must, because our souls are deeply akin, because even when we are apart our joint work unites us.[73]

Other parallels occurred. Just as Jung imagined himself especially chosen by God in his Basel Cathedral revelation, Spielrein too thought of herself as having a "higher calling". Perhaps, she speculated, it came from her grandfather

[68] To Freud, 21 June 1909, in McGuire p. 236.

[69] Diary entry, 21 September 1909, in Carotenuto p. 6.

[70] Diary entry, 23 September 1909, ibid. p. 8.

[71] Diary entry 9 September 1910, ibid. p. 8.

[72] Diary entry 11 September 1910, ibid. p. 12.

[73] Diary entry, *circa* September 1910, ibid. p. 20.

and great-grandfather both being rabbis and hence "God's elect".[74] Jung later described this insight as a product of her analysis with him. Initially, he said, "All her conscious activity was directed towards flirtation, clothes, and sex, because she knew of nothing else. She knew only the intellect and lived a meaningless life". But then it became clear, he went on, that "[i]n reality she was a child of God whose destiny was to fulfill His secret will". He had therefore "had to awaken mythological and religious ideas in her, for she belonged to that class of human beings of whom spiritual activity is demanded. Thus her life took on a meaning, and no trace of the neurosis was left".[75]

Jung was drawn to her by their spiritual similarity. Spielrein again wrote of "poetry" between them, adding "He said then that he loves me because of the remarkable parallelism in our thoughts".[76] But their time together was running out. In January 1911 she took her final exams. She defended her dissertation on 9 February, and a couple of days later left Zurich for Munich. But she remained on Jung's mind. Writing favourably about her dissertation to Freud, Jung said the case of schizophrenia on which it was based demonstrated the need "to bring to light the inner world produced by the introversion of libido, which in paranoia suddenly appears in distorted form as a delusional system".[77] In this Spielrein had undoubtedly been inspired by Jung, as he was by her, in their ideas on the beneficial effects of psychoanalysis as means of transforming libido and love.

Transformations

The first part of Jung's book, *Transformations and Symbols of the Libido*, was published as an essay in the IPA journal in mid-August 1911. Freud who, arguably inspired by Jung, was now writing his first book about religion, *Totem and Taboo*, told Jung of his eagerness to read his transformations essay.[78] It began with Jung's already announced theory of two types of thinking. Borrowing William James' terms,[79] Jung described logical thinking as "directed" and "adapted to reality", symbolic thinking as "non-directed" and "merely associative". It is "guided by unconscious motives", he said, by "primitive or archaic thought-forms".[80]

74 Diary entry, 18 October 1910, ibid. p. 21.

75 Jung 1961 p. 162.

76 Diary entry, 9 November 1910, in Carotenuto p. 33.

77 To Freud, 12 June 1911, in McGuire pp. 426–7.

78 To Jung, 20 August 1911, ibid. p. 438.

79 From W. James (1890) *The Principles of Psychology, Vol.II*, Boston: Dover, 1950, pp. 330, 325.

80 C. G. Jung (1911–12) *Symbols of Transformation*, **CW5** pp. 18, 28.

Jung illustrated symbolic thinking with a case published in 1906 by William James' spiritualist researcher friend, Theodore Flournoy. The case concerned a young American woman, Miss Daisy Miller, who, having fallen in love with a naval officer she had seen in the port of Catania in Sicily found herself doing automatic writing on the journey taking her, via Naples, to Lausanne. Her automatic writing resulted in a poem beginning "when God had first made sound", and in another "hypnagogic" poem and play. They in turn evoked various associations – a "kaleidoscope", she said, of fragments – associations to Milton's *Paradise Lost*, *The Book of Job*, Haydn's *Creation* oratorio, Shakespeare's *Julius Caesar*, the story of Buddha leaving his father's home, Samuel Johnson's *Rasselas*, Longfellow's *Song of Hiawatha*, and Wagner's *Siegfried*.[81]

From all this Jung concluded that Miller's automatic writings were examples of ways in which sexual love, the libido, or what Jung called "psychic energy" can be transformed into what Jung called "the god-image". This transformation is effected, he said, through use of "archetypal patterns" surfacing, as expressed by Miss Miller, in the work of Shakespeare, Milton, Johnson, Wagner, and so on. These patterns, said Jung, lead us to worship the spirit – or psychic force – within us as "something divine".[82] Spielrein wrote something similar in her dissertation. It too concerned what could be called transformations and symbols of the libido. Specifically it concerned a Protestant woman married to a Catholic who suffered with what Spielrein called a "Catholicizing complex". Spielrein conceptualized her treatment of the woman's schizophrenia as entailing transforming this complex through what Spielrein referred to as "mythological" and "Sistine" experiments into ideas about poetry and art as synonyms for religion.[83]

Spielrein's dissertation was published in the same August issue of the IPA journal as Jung's account of Daisy Miller. At the next month's IPA conference in Weimar, Jung argued that thinking in terms of age-old universal images or symbols is particularly characteristic of schizophrenia.[84] Freud reiterated the point at the same conference. The case of Schreber, he said, proved that:

> Jung had excellent grounds for his assertion that the mythopeic forces of mankind are not extinct, but that to this very day they give rise in the neuroses to the same psychical products as in the remote past ages.[85]

....

81 F. Miller (1906) Quelques faits d'imagination créatrice subconsciente, *Archives de Psychologie*, 5 pp. 36–51, in **CW5** pp. 447–62, 454.

82 Jung 1911–12 p. 86.

83 S. Spielrein (1911) On the psychological content of a case of schizophrenia (Dementia Praecox), in Kerr pp. 296–7, see also S. Spielrein (1912) Destruction as a cause of coming into being, *Journal of Analytical Psychology*, 1994 (April), **39** (2) pp. 155–86.

84 C. Jung (1911) Contributions to symbolism, **CW18** p. 446 (abstract by Rank).

85 S. Freud (1912) Postscript [to the Schreber case], **SE12** pp. 80–2, 81.

Soon after, however, Freud also cautioned Jung against extending the meaning of the libido. It means nothing more nor less, he insisted, than "the power behind the sexual drive".[86]

But Jung persisted in extending the meaning of the libido. In the second part of his *Transformations* book – based, his wife Emma told Freud, on his "self-analysis"[87] – Jung repeatedly quoted Spielrein's dissertation in his support. He quoted, for instance, her account of symbols originating in "the striving of a complex for dissolution in the common totality of thought" so as to lose "its personal quality". He also drew on her notion of symbolic "dissolution or transformation" as "mainspring of poetry, painting, and every form of art".[88] He cited her observation of her schizophrenic patient using symbols of sacrificial death, resurrection, and regeneration including an image of the snake. Jung called it "God's animal, it has such wonderful colours . . . it can have divine judgement . . . would save the children who are needed to preserve human life". In the same way, he said, Daisy Miller's hypnagogic fantasy of a snake symbolized "the unconscious psyche of the author herself".[89]

Most of all, however, the second part of Jung's *Transformations* book, first published in the IPA journal in February 1912, dwelt on the symbol of the hero struggling to be reborn and freed from the mother. Again Jung wrote to Spielrein about the similarity of their ideas. Unconsciously, he said, they had "swallowed" part of each other's souls. But, he went on, this "secret penetration of thoughts" must not become public.[90] For the moment Freud too swallowed Jung's ideas. In a preface to an essay published that March he wrote approvingly of the report of one of Jung's students, Johann Honegger, that, as Freud put it

> The fantasies of certain mental patients (*dementia praecox*) coincided strikingly with the mythological cosmogonies of ancient peoples of whom these uneducated patients could not possibly have had any scholarly knowledge.[91]

But Jung criticized Freud. He criticized his claim that religion is a defence against an Oedipal wish to murder one's father and marry one's mother. The

---

86 To Jung, 30 November 1911, in McGuire p. 469.

87 To Freud, 14 November 1911, ibid. p. 462.

88 Jung 1911–12 p. 141.

89 Ibid. p. 437.

90 To Spielrein, 25 March 1912, in Kerr p. 403.

91 W. McGuire (1991) Introduction, *Psychology of the Unconscious: A Study of the Transformations and Symbolisms of the LIbid.o*, London: Routledge, pp. xvii–xxxii, xxiii.

mythological significance of the mother, he insisted, far outweighs what Freud called "the biological incest problem".[92]

Spielrein now met Freud, in April 1912, and discussed with him the possibility of his taking her on for analysis that autumn.[93] Whether or not Jung knew this, he was hurt by Freud telling him that he would be visiting Jung's erstwhile Burghölzli colleague, Ludwig Binswanger, the next day in Kreuzlinger, in North East Switzerland, but would not have time to see Jung. Jung concluded that this was because Freud objected to his "interpretation of the incest concept" and "development of the libido theory".[94] Freud tried to reassure him. But he only made matters worse by implying that, like Adler, Jung too was defecting from psychoanalysis.

Jung was indeed increasingly departing from Freud's theories. Shortly after Spielrein's marriage that summer to a Russian doctor, Paul Scheftel, Jung gave lectures in a small Catholic university, Fordham, in New York. Recounting them to Freud following his return to Europe, Jung said:

> Naturally I also made room for those of my views which deviate in places from the hitherto existing conceptions, particularly in regard to the libido theory. I found that my version of psychoanalysis won over many people who until now had been put off by the problem of sexuality in neurosis.[95]

Freud was annoyed by Jung thus disposing of sex in telling Americans about his theory. Emphasizing the point, he began his next letter to him frostily, "Dear Doctor", not "Dear Friend" as before.[96]

Ten days later the situation was aggravated at a psychoanalytic meeting in Munich. Freud complained that the Swiss failed to credit him in their psychoanalytic publications. Jung likened this to the history of Amenhotep, credited with introducing monotheism into Egypt and in doing so, eliminating the name of his father and of others as gods. "[T]he father already has a name", Jung explained, "whereas the son must go out and make one for himself".[97] At this Freud fainted as he had at their meeting in Bremen three years before. He told the British psychoanalyst, Ernest Jones, that his fainting was due to "homosexual feeling" rekindled by his first having been to Munich to see Fliess when he was ill there in 1894.[98] He also told Jones, "You are right in supposing

92 To Freud, 27 April 1912, in McGuire p. 502.

93 R. Hayman (1999) *A Life of Jung*, London: Bloomsbury, p. xiv.

94 To Freud, 8 June 1912, in McGuire p. 509.

95 To Freud, 11 November 1912, ibid. p. 515.

96 To Jung, 14 November 1912, ibid. p. 517.

97 In Kerr p. 429.

98 To Jones, 8 December 1912, in P. Gay (1988) *Freud*, London: Macmillan, p. 276.

that I had transferred to Jung homosex[ual] feelings from another part but I am glad to find that I have no difficulty in removing them for free circulation".[99] Remove them he did. A few days later he wrote to Jung suggesting they end their friendship. Jung immediately agreed saying "I never thrust my friendship on anyone", adding, like Hamlet, "The rest is silence".[100]

As it turned out Jung's Fordham lectures did not depart as much from Freud's theory as Freud had feared. In them Jung recommended adopting Freud's method in the initial stages of therapy so as to discover the patient's history and wishful fantasies through analysing the patient's dreams. But, Jung went on, it is also necessary to consider the "teleological and prospective significance" of the unconscious revealed by the patient's dreams. This is necessary, he said, to enable the patient to move out of what he called "the semi-infantile transference relationship" with the analyst into a life chosen by the patient himself. Its symbolic direction, he said, could be very much enhanced by studying mythology.[101]

Jung now renamed his approach to therapy "analytical psychology" in a lecture in London on 5 August 1913. In his lecture he also argued against Freud that dreams are not caused by sex. Rather, he argued, dreams use sex as "a means of expression".[102] Nor is their aim to fulfill a sexual wish. Treatment entails discovering the meaning of the patients' dreams so as to help guide them from the past and their inner world to the future. "For me", Jung said, "the dream is, in the first instance, a subliminal picture of the actual psychological situation of the individual in his waking state".[103] Pursuing the dream's symbolic meaning without reducing it to sex, he maintained, cultivates a psychological attitude that is as important to freeing the neurotic from his illness as the help "primitive man" derived from "religious and philosophical symbols".[104] Analytical psychology, Jung therefore argued, in another lecture in London the next week, gives centrality not to sex but to the spirit, to the libido understood as "vital energy . . . élan vital".[105]

Soon after, in his September 1913 preface to *Totem and Taboo*, Freud differentiated his approach from that of Jung in his 1912 and 1913 transformations essays. The atmosphere between them at their next and last meeting the same

[99] To Jones, 26 December 1912, ibid. p. 276.

[100] To Freud, 6 January 1913, in McGuire p. 540.

[101] C. G. Jung (1913) The theory of psychoanalysis, CW4 pp. 83–226, 201, 203.

[102] C. G. Jung (1913) General aspects of psychoanalysis, CW4 pp. 229–42, 238.

[103] Ibid. p. 240.

[104] Ibid. p. 241.

[105] C. G. Jung (1913) Psychoanalysis and neurosis, CW4 pp. 243–51, 247, 248.

month at a conference in Munich was, apparently, "disagreeable".[106] Feelings between them were presumably not improved by the paper Jung presented at this conference. In it he put forward for the first time his theory of "extrovert" and "introvert" personality types. He allied it to a distinction made by William James between "tender-minded" and "tough-minded" or, as Jung put it, between "spiritually-minded" and "materially-minded".[107] Freud and Adler, Jung indicated, were both materially-minded – Freud in emphasizing sex, Adler in emphasizing power.

Divided from Freud, Jung was now also further divided from Spielrein who gave birth later that month to her first child, Renate. Soon afterwards Jung broke down. On a railway journey to Schaffhausen in October he suffered a terrifying hallucination. "I saw the mighty yellow waves, the floating rubble of civilization, and the drowned bodies of uncounted thousands", he said. "Then the whole sea turned to blood".[108] Two weeks later the terrifying hallucinations returned. Perhaps fear of going mad contributed to a somewhat paranoid letter he wrote at about this time to Freud saying that, since he had heard from one of his Zurich colleagues, Maeder, that Freud doubted his good faith, and since this made continuing collaboration between them impossible, he was resigning as editor of the IPA journal.[109]

Jung now became increasingly immersed in his hallucinations. At first he resisted pursuing them for fear, as he put it, "of losing command . . . and becoming a prey to the fantasies".[110] But, on 12 December 1913, he decided to pursue and sink into them whereupon, he said, "I plunged down into dark depths".[111] His fantasies included dreaming, six nights later, of killing Wagner's hero, Siegfried. He was full of remorse. Perhaps, suggests one commentator,[112] this was due to guilt at betraying Spielrein's Siegfried-complex love of him, and to unhappiness at Freud rejecting him, thereby thwarting Jung's ambition to become son and heroic heir to the psychoanalysis Freud had founded.

Jung now turned from outward heroics to inner fantasies. He was helped, he said, by imagining "a steep descent" into them.[113] He gave up his outer

---

[106] Jones quoted in McGuire p. 550.

[107] W. James (1907) *Pragmatism*, Cambridge: Harvard University Press, 1975 p. 13 in C. G. Jung (1913) A contribution to the study of psychological types, **CW6** pp. 499–509, 502.

[108] Jung 1961 p. 199.

[109] To Freud, 27 October 1913, in McGuire p. 550.

[110] Jung 1961 p. 202.

[111] Ibid. p. 203.

[112] Kerr.

[113] Jung 1961 p. 205.

commitments. He resigned from his lectureship at Zurich University. In the same month, April 1914, he also resigned as president of the IPA, from which the Zurich Psycho-Analytic Society had seceded ten days earlier. "So we are rid of them at last", Freud wrote to Karl Abraham, who had once worked with Jung at the Burghölzli, "the brutal holy Jung and his pious parrots".[114]

That July the IPA journal carried two articles by Freud criticizing Jung and Swiss psychoanalysis generally. In the first article,[115] Freud took issue with Jung's long-standing dissent from his sexual theory as regards schizophrenia. In contrast with Jung, Freud argued that schizophrenia, like other mental illness, involves sex and love, specifically regression from sexual love of others to narcissistic love of oneself. Developmentally, Freud argued, this narcissistic self-love is the successor to the child's first part-object sexual love for his mother's breast, and for his own mouth, fingers, anus, faeces, and genitals. Schizophrenia, insisted Freud, involves regression to whole-object, narcissistic self-love, not transformation of the libido, as Jung claimed, into heightened interest in the divine.

In his second article, Freud criticized Jung's boast that he had won over many in America to psychoanalysis through reducing its emphasis on sex. In doing so, Freud implied, Jung had not merely altered psychoanalysis, he had completely abandoned and betrayed it. He had given up individual psychology for anthropology, and the biological reality of sex for symbolic abstraction. In Jung's system, Freud wrote,

> For sexual libido an abstract concept has been substituted . . . The Oedipus complex has a merely "symbolic" meaning: the mother in it means the unattainable, which must be renounced in the interests of civilization; the father who is killed in the Oedipus myth is the "inner" father, from whom one must set oneself free in order to become independent.[116]

Jung wrongly attended, said Freud, less to the past of his patients than to the present and to generalities about their future "life-task". Freud illustrated the point by quoting a patient who described his experience of Jungian analysis as dismissing transference-love as merely a "libidinal symbol", and as instead urging "inward concentration" through "religious meditation".[117]

To all this Freud added that Jung wrongly equated consciously remembered dreams with their unconscious content. Jung thereby overlooked the process by which through the dream-work the unconscious is defended against and

---

[114] To Abraham, 26 July 1914, in Gay p. 241.

[115] S. Freud (1914) On narcissism, **SE14** pp. 73–102.

[116] S. Freud (1914) On the history of the psycho-analytic movement, **SE14** pp. 7–66, 62.

[117] Ibid. p. 63.

repressively disguised. Undoing this defence through attending to their patients' free associations to details of their dreams reveals that dreams are not simply a means of solving life tasks suggested by the therapist. Nor, Freud went on, is the sexual content of dreams and neurotic symptoms simply an archaic mode of symbolic expression. Rather mental illness is due to sexual interest being withdrawn from outer to inner reality. It is this withdrawal of, and defence against sexual interest that needs addressing in analysis. Sex and love cannot be freed from what Jung called the patient's "complexes" through simply urging patients to sublimate their urge for love and sex through transforming it into symbols.

Jung nevertheless continued to pursue this aim in analysis. Beginning work at 7.30 in the morning, he saw patients up to three times a week in face-to-face analysis, unlike Freud who saw patients six days a week, with the patient out of direct eye-contact lying on a couch. Jung also altered Freud's method, supplementing Freud's talking cure approach to analysis by encouraging his patients to write down, paint, and draw the figures emerging in their free associations. An example was Fanny Bowditch Katz (an early follower of Jung). Describing her drawing in analysis with Jung, she said, he taught her that she should "learn to understand them and how each of them can be lived". He also taught her, she said, "the value and importance of recognizing one's archaic tendencies as part of oneself – loving them as being a part of one's soul".[118]

Jung did much the same in his own self-analysis. By 1915 his own mental health had become so precarious that his wife, Emma, agreed to his then mistress, Toni Wolff, sometimes living with them.[119] But Jung continued to be beset by visions. He also felt he had lost his "soul" to the "land of the dead".[120] He deduced that such experiences are the source of the dead returning in spiritualist seances. He described this in a book, *Seven Sermons to the Dead*, which was privately printed and published in 1916.[121] By then he was also painting mandalas (see e.g. Fig. 3.1).[122] That autumn he again wrote of the importance of attending to visual images, as well as to patients' verbal free associations, in therapy. Rather

---

[118] In F. Katz, 15 February 1915, in R. Hayman (1999) *A Life of Jung*, London: Bloomsbury, p. 193.

[119] Kerr p. 503.

[120] Jung 1961 p. 216.

[121] Subsequently included as an appendix to the second edition of *Memories, Dreams, Reflections* – see **CW18** p. 663 n. 4.

[122] Mandala of a Modern Man, in C. G. Jung (1959) *The Archetypes and the Collective Unconscious*, **CW9i** frontispiece.

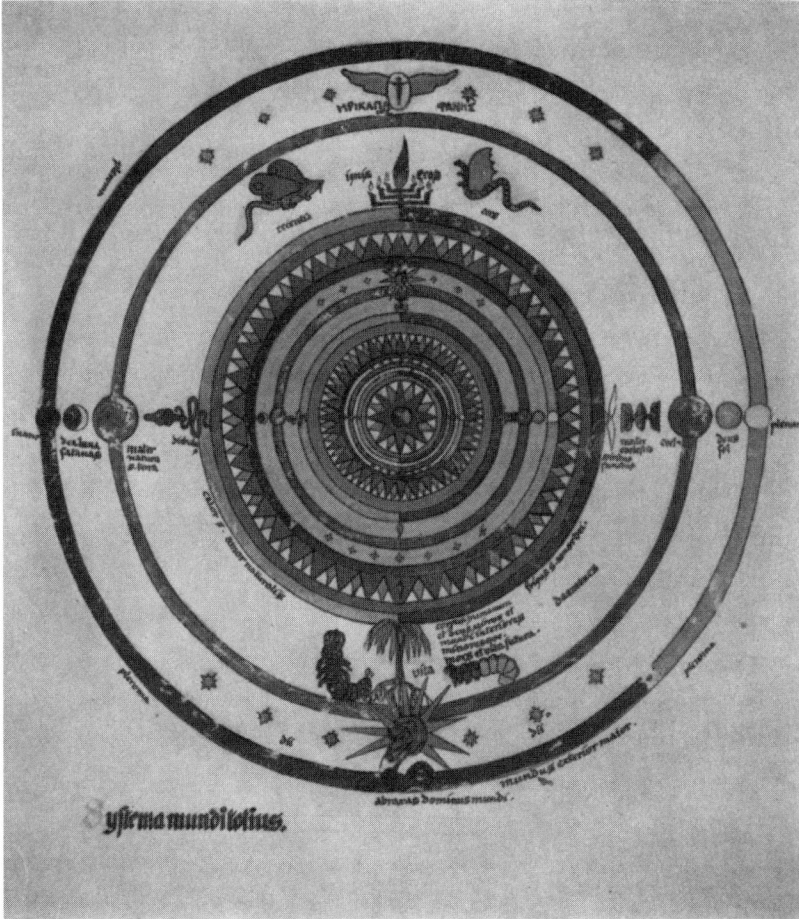

Fig. 3.1 Mandala of a Modern Man – C.G. Jung.

than reduce either to biology and sex, he urged patients to use them constructively to discover their meaning.

He also recommended patients to attend to their spontaneously occurring daydreams. In being more coherent and composed than our sleeping dreams, he argued, daydreams lend themselves more readily to the therapeutic task of synthesis and construction. Jung accordingly recommended patients to let themselves sink into whatever mood they found themselves in, and to note whatever daydreams, fantasies, and associations occurred. They might emerge as pictures the patient could draw or paint, or as voices or words the patient could write. Either way, said Jung, patients can thereby realize "the transcendent function", which he defined as the bringing together of consciousness with the transcendence of the unconscious. Patients could thereby become free from dependence on the therapist through discovering what Jung called "the courage" to be themselves.[123]

In a lecture published in 1917 Jung rooted transcendence in what he now for the first time called "the collective unconscious". He described it as composed of "impersonal . . . inherited categories".[124] Health, he said, entails "individuation", reconnecting with both one's personal and collective unconscious. In her 1907 essay about transformation (see p. 70) Spielrein had written about losing oneself in another in sexual love. Jung now wrote of this in relation to God. In loving another, he wrote, the lover:

> Gives his supreme good, his love, not to the soul but to a human being who stands for his soul, and from this human being it goes to God and through this human being it comes back to the lover, but only so long as this human being stands for his soul. . . . Thus I, as an individual, can discharge my collective function either by giving my love to the soul and so procuring the ransom I owe to society, or, as a lover, by loving the human being through whom I receive the gift of God.[125]

Jung later attributed his recovery from his breakdown during the First World War to the intervention of just such a loved and loving intermediary. He called her his "anima". He described her as a woman patient returning as a voice telling him that what he was doing was art. She had, he said, "become a living figure" in his mind. In writing down the fantasies occurring to him during his breakdown, he said, he was "in effect writing letters" to her.[126]

Perhaps the patient was Sabina. Towards the end of the war she wrote to him from Lausanne about his recently published theory of the collective unconscious,[127] and followed this with further letters dwelling on the "subconscious". She distinguished it from the repressed unconscious and described it as consisting of universal "subliminal symbols . . . more archaic than the corresponding conscious thoughts".[128] Early the next year she wrote to Jung about her symbol of Siegfried during her analysis with him:

> In the beginning Siegfried was probably "real" for my subconscious . . . I was still much too young, and my first love and "vocation" were too sacred for me to follow your arguments and give heed to the symbols that the subconscious probably produced to warn me.[129]

---

[123]   C. G. Jung (1916) The transcendent function, CW8 pp. 76–91, 91.

[124]   C. G. Jung (1917) *On the Psychology of the Unconscious*, CW7 pp. 127–241, 138.

[125]   C. G. Jung (1916) Adaptation, individuation, collectivity, **CW18** pp. 449–454, 453–54.

[126]   Jung 1961 pp. 210–12.

[127]   To Jung, 27 November 1917, in Carotenuto p. 50.

[128]   To Jung, 20 December 1917, ibid. p. 62.

[129]   To Jung, 6 January 1918, ibid. p. 77.

Siegfried, wrote Jung, was "a godlike part of herself". She should accept him as such. With Siegfried, Jung told her, "I lit in you a new light that you must safeguard for times of darkness".[130] Soon Jung rooted this light or spirit in what he called "archetypes" of the collective unconscious.

Jung first introduced the term "archetype" into his theoretical system in a lecture in Bedford College in London in July 1919. Together with the instincts, he said, archetypes constitute "the collective unconscious". Archetypes, he said, are "inborn forms of 'intuition'". They are "necessary *a priori* determinants of all psychic processes".[131] Meanwhile, still in correspondence with Sabina who, following her husband's return to Russia in 1915, remained alone with their daughter in Lausanne, Jung told her of her love inspiring his discovery of the collective unconscious and its archetypes:

> The love of S. for J. made the latter aware of something he had previously only vaguely suspected, that is, of a power in the unconscious that shapes one's destiny, a power which later led him to things of the greatest importance. The relationship had to be "sublimated" because otherwise it would have led him to delusion and madness (the concretization of the unconscious).[132]

Jung now increasingly came to relate this "power" to God. During the war he had described an "ineradicable substrate of the human mind" which he then said was knowable through the idea of God. Jung called this idea the "God-image". He said it corresponds "to a definite complex of psychological factors" that psychology could and should take into account.[133] After the war Jung described God, as opposed to our idea of God, as an "unconscious content" or archetype of the collective unconscious. When withdrawn from projection into others, he said, it gives rise to an inward "feeling of intense vitality" and a sense of "oneness of being . . . between conscious and unconscious".[134]

Detailing this in his book, *Psychological Types*, Jung also detailed the archetype of the anima. In contrast with the outward directed "persona", he said, the anima (or animus in women) is an inwardly directed "soul-image". When projected into another, he said, it makes them into an "object of intense love or equally intense hate (or fear)". It is the stuff of falling in love. "Wherever an impassioned, almost magical, relationship exists between the sexes", he wrote, "it is invariably a question of a projected soul-image".[135] This soul-image, or

---

130 To Spielrein, 3 April 1919, in Kerr p. 491.

131 C. G. Jung (1919) Instinct and the unconscious, **CW8** pp. 129–38, 133.

132 To Spielrein, 1 September 1919, in Carotenuto p. 190.

133 C. G. Jung (1916) General aspects of dream psychology, **CW8** pp. 237–80, 278, 279.

134 C. G. Jung (1921) *Psychological Types*, **CW6** pp. 247–48.

135 Ibid. p. 471.

anima, he later wrote, is "the archetype of life itself" without which existence remains meaningless "chaotic capriciousness", mere "aimless experience".[136]

Psychological Types was published in 1921. Two years later Jung's mother died. Soon after he began building a retreat for himself, at Bollingen, near his family home in Küsnach. He also travelled widely – to Tunisia, New Mexico, Mombassa, and elsewhere – collecting evidence of the universality of the symbols and archetypes of the collective unconscious. He also related them to the transformations sought in the past by alchemy and in the present through religion and therapy.

Religion and therapy

In 1927, as we have seen, Freud dismissed religion as founded on illusion. Jung, by contrast, in an essay the next year, recommended religion. He approved of the way that, in Catholicism, what he called the "contents" of the collective unconscious and its archetypes, and what Catholicism calls "grace", are mediated by the priest hearing and asking questions about the penitent's confession. By contrast, Jung noted, Protestants lack any such personal intermediary. They are left with the responsibility of discovering their soul – the contents of their unconscious, their God – for themselves. Protestant pastors, therefore, knowing that their task is "the cure of souls", and knowing that moralizing will only strengthen the forces of repression, accordingly look, claimed Jung, to analytical psychology where, as he put it, "soul must work on soul", analyst and patient together in an "I/Thou" relationship, just as in the interchange of priest and penitent in the Catholic confessional.[137]

Jung detailed this further in a lecture in 1929. In his lecture he described four stages of analytical therapy. Since, he said, a major source of distress bringing people to analysis arises from secrets they keep from themselves and others, analysis should begin with confession. He called this first stage "catharsis". He likened this stage's attention to the patient's dreams and free associations to the meditation and contemplation practiced in yoga as means of getting in touch with the "hinterland", as he put it, of one's mind. But, Jung noted, confession in analysis becomes obstructed by the patient's transference onto the analyst of their relationships as children with their parents. This leads to the second stage of analysis. It is concerned, said Jung, with the "elucidation" of the transference. Freud described this elucidation as involving interpreting and

---

[136] C. G. Jung (1934) *Archetypes of the Collective Unconscious*, **CW9i** pp. 3–41, 32.
[137] C. G. Jung (1928) Psychoanalysis and the cure of souls, **CW11** pp. 348–54, 350, 351, 353.

putting the patient's unconscious fantasies, transferred onto the therapist, into words so they can become more fully conscious.

To Freud's method Jung added two further stages – "education" and "transformation". Both stages, he said, entail the patient and therapist becoming aware of their influence on each other. Whereas Freud advised psychoanalysts (as in his June 1907 letter to Jung about his analytic involvement with Spielrein) to harden themselves against the counter-transference impact of their patients on them, Jung emphasized the reverse. Perhaps drawing on the transformation brought about in both him and Spielrein by her love, Jung emphasized that it is just as important for analysts to be open to being influenced by the patient as it is for the patient to be open to being influenced by the analyst. This is crucial, he said, to the education stage of analysis enabling the patient to learn from its previous two stages what to do next.

Mutual recognition by patients and therapists of their impact on each other is also crucial, said Jung, to the fourth – "transformation" – stage of analysis. Just like the patient, the doctor too, maintained Jung, "is equally a part of the psychic process of treatment and therefore equally exposed to the transforming influences". The doctor, added Jung, "must change himself if he is to become capable of changing the patient".[138] This entails the doctor or therapist, as well as the patient, facing "things in his own nature". It entails them facing aspects of themselves that they might not want to face, aspects which, as Jung put it, "are utterly opposed to normalization, or which continue to haunt him [the analyst] in the most distressing way".[139]

In another essay he emphasized encouraging patients to describe their dreams in as much detail as possible so as to discover how they compensate for what is conscious. This is further helped, he argued, by taking into account the dreamer's specific philosophical, moral, and religious convictions.[140] He talked more about religion at a conference in Strasbourg in May 1932. In his talk he rejected the emphasis of Freud and Adler on biological and social instincts of sex and power. For, he argued, instincts themselves have no meaning. Focusing on them is therefore hardly appropriate in seeking to treat the feelings of meaninglessness which he believed were often the main cause of older people, at least, seeking psychotherapy. Nor, he said, is it any good the priest, pastor, or doctor condemning those who come to them for help, their sexual proclivities, for instance, as sinful. People can only begin to recover a

---

[138] C. G. Jung (1929) Problems of modern psychotherapy, **CW**16 pp. 53–75, 72, 73.

[139] Ibid. pp. 73–74.

[140] C. G. Jung (1931) The practical use of dream-analysis, **CW**16 pp. 139–61.

sense of meaning and wholeness in their lives, Jung argued, through accepting what they otherwise split off and reject in themselves. This depends, he continued, on those from whom they seek help accepting what they can least accept in themselves. Or, as he put it, "the patient does not feel himself accepted unless the very worst in him is accepted too".[141]

Penitents, parishioners, and patients can only feel fully accepted by the priests, pastors, or therapists they consult provided the latter fully accept themselves. This too includes accepting what is least acceptable in themselves. It depends for all of us, wrote Jung, on facing and becoming conscious of "the shadow-side and the evil within us". Nor can we do this alone. It depends on spiritual help without which, wrote Jung, we cannot withstand "the powers of darkness".[142] In this help comes not only from personal involvement with another – with a priest, pastor, or therapist. It also comes, said Jung, from impersonal archetypes within the collective unconscious. Describing the therapeutic effects of these archetypes, he said:

> It is as though, at the climax of the illness, the destructive powers were converted into healing forces. This is brought about by the archetypes awaking to independent life and taking over the guidance of the psychic personality, thus supplanting the ego with its futile willing and striving. As a religious-minded person would say: guidance has come from God.

Such appeals to submission to higher authority were now becoming commonplace with the rise of Fascism in Germany. In May 1933 the Nazis burnt freethinking books, such as those of Freud. The next month, in a radio broadcast, Jung weighed in on the side of the Nazis in criticizing Freud. The novelist, Thomas Mann, whose books had also been burnt, took issue with Jung, saying "Anyone in these times who wallows in 'soul' is old-fashioned both intellectually and morally".[143] Jung nevertheless continued his soul-wallowing. He gave a talk that summer about yoga and meditation at an Eranos conference organized in a spiritual centre near Ascona by Lake Maggiore in Italy. And he arguably collaborated with the Nazis both in chairing the 1934 and 1935 annual congresses of the General Medical Society for Psychotherapy, and in appointing Göring's cousin as co-editor of the society's journal, *Zentralblatt*.

In 1935 Jung also gave lectures at the Tavistock Clinic in London. In them he described for the first time as "active imagination" his method of visual association, based, he said, on the fact that "when we concentrate on an inner

---

[141] C. G. Jung (1932) Psychotherapists or the clergy, **CW11** pp. 327–47, 338.

[142] Ibid. pp. 343–44.

[143] In Hayman p. 319.

picture and when we are careful not to interrupt the natural flow of events, our unconscious will produce a series of images which make a complete story".[144] Two years later he gave the Terry Lectures in Yale. In them he described this process in religious terms. He described religious experience as emanating from what he called "a dynamic agency or effect not caused by an arbitrary act of will" which, he said, "seizes and controls . . . the subject independent of his will".[145] Extending this to therapy, he argued that therapists should enable those seeking their help to take seriously the forces of their personal and collective unconscious, the latter expressing itself through symbols revealing what he called "the God within" us.[146]

To illustrate the point, he cited the case of a lapsed Catholic, demoralized by neurosis, who, through pursuing his dreams arrived at a vision of two circles with a common centre which he understood as "the world clock". It gave him, he said, "an impression of the most sublime harmony".[147] Jung interpreted it as a mandala. It expressed, he said, "the union of the soul with God", psychic wholeness, "the self", which Jung defined as the sum total of consciousness unified with the transcendent unconscious.[148]

Jung gave the Terry Lectures in 1937. At the end of that year he went to India. Here, he later reported, he had a dream which convinced him he should devote himself to studying the history, traditions, symbols and rituals of Christianity. He also wrote about eastern and western mysticism. He wrote about Indian religion shifting its practitioners' centre of gravity from the outer-directed ego to the inner-directed self. He dubbed this outer–inner shift a movement "from man to God".[149] In 1939 he also wrote about Buddhism.[150] The next August, however, he returned to Christianity with an Eranos lecture about the symbolism of the Trinity;[151] the following May, he lectured about the transformation of spirit into matter symbolized in the Eucharist and Mass.[152]

....

144 C. G. Jung (1935) The Tavistock Lectures, **CW18** pp. 5–182, 6, 172.

145 C. G. Jung (1937) *Psychology and Religion*, **CW11** pp. 1–105, 7.

146 Ibid. p. 58.

147 Ibid. pp. 65, 72.

148 Ibid. pp. 72, 82.

149 C. G. Jung (1944) The holy men of India, **CW10** pp. 578–86, 581.

150 C. G. Jung (1939) Psychological commentary on *The Tibetan Book of the Great Liberation*, **CW11** pp. 475–508, 482.

151 C. G. Jung (1940) On the psychology of the idea of the Trinity, expanded in C. G. Jung (1948) A psychological approach to the dogma of the Trinity, **CW11** pp. 107–200.

152 C. G. Jung (1940/41) Transformation symbolism in the Mass, **CW11** pp. 201–96.

Not long after, in 1942, Sabina Spielrein was killed with her daughters (Renate and Eva, born 1926) during the German occupation of Rostov-on-Don, where she had returned in 1924.[153] Sabina was Jewish. Not so Jung. At the end of the war he became increasingly interested in Catholicism. In 1945 a Catholic priest, Victor White, who had read his 1928 essay, "Psychoanalysis and the cure of souls", sent Jung his writing about religion. Jung was delighted by White's planned extension of analytical psychology to what Jung called "ecclesiastical doctrine".[154] Jung's own extension of analytical psychology now included likening the doctrine of Christ on the cross to the patient in therapy at a crossroads between what he is and has "no wish to be". Jung called the latter "the shadow".[155] He wrote more about Christ and God in subsequent books and papers. He also welcomed the inclusion, in November 1950, of a female figure – the Virgin Mary – in the Catholic pantheon,[156] just as he had himself included a female figure – the anima – in the pantheon of archetypes he ascribed to the collective unconscious.

But in rooting the anima and God in the unconscious, Jung overlooked the separateness of God. Following the 1951 publication of his book, *Aion*, dwelling on parallels between the transformations of Christian and alchemical symbolism, the Jewish theologian, Martin Buber, criticized Jung on this account. He quoted Jung describing religion as "a living relationship to psychical events which do not depend upon consciousness but instead take place on the other side of it in the darkness of the psychical hinterland".[157] With this Jung did away with God as "the eternal thou".[158] He reduced religious experience, said Buber, from transcendence to immanence. Or, as Buber also put it,

> More precisely, it [Jung's analytical psychology] is not the relation of an I to a Thou. That is, however, the way in which the unmistakably religious of all ages have understood their religion even if they longed most intensely to let their I be mystically absorbed into the Thou.[159]

---

[153] Where her husband became incurably insane in the early 1930s and later died of a heart attack. For further details about Spielrein's work see J. Sayers (in press) Transforming at-one-ment, *Psychoanalysis and History*.

[154] To White, 5 October 1945, in Hayman p. 386.

[155] C. G. Jung (1946) *The Psychology of the Transference*, **CW**16 pp. 163–323, 262.

[156] e.g. C. G. Jung (1952) *Answer to Job*, **CW**11 pp. 355–470, 458 n. 4.

[157] M. Buber (1952) Religion and modern thinking, reprinted in *Eclipse of God*, New York: Harper & Row, pp. 63–92, 79.

[158] See e.g. M. Buber (1923) *I and Thou*, New York: Scribner, 1987, p. 100.

[159] Buber 1952 p. 79.

Buber's critique of Jung was published in February 1952. Three months later Jung wrote a foreword to Victor White's book, *God and the Unconscious*. The same year Jung's book, *Answer to Job*, was published. In it Jung described the Jewish God, Yahweh, being transformed through a woman character, Sophia, enabling him to become conscious of the wrong he had done Job in making a Faustian pact with the devil allowing him to plague Job. In enabling him to become conscious of this wrong, Sophia enabled Yahweh to become conscious of the need to atone for it by becoming a man like Job. This in turn led to God's answer to Job, concluded Jung, through Himself as Christ crying out, "My God, my God, why hast thou forsaken me?" For then God became aware, said Jung, of what it is to be mortal and suffer. Man, in the form of Christ, thereby also became God.

With his book about Job, Jung in a sense answered Buber by emphasizing that it is through others – through Sophia's intercession, and through God's loving identification with Christ on the cross – that one becomes transformed into becoming one with God. But now Victor White took issue with Jung. In 1955 he wrote criticizing Jung's notion of God as "Evil" as regards Job.[160] With this they stopped being friends. The ending of their friendship left Jung again alone as he had been as a child. His First World War mistress, Toni Wolff, had died a couple of years before, on 19 March 1953. His wife, Emma, died on 27 November 1955. Undaunted by isolation, and by White's criticism, however, Jung reiterated in his autobiography, begun in 1957, the existence of both good and evil in God. He also reiterated in a BBC television interview in October 1959 his notion of God as existing within us, within what he called "an impersonal stratum in our psyche".[161]

In September 1960 he became ill and died the following year, on 6 June 1961. His autobiography, *Memories, Dreams, Reflections*, was published soon after. Reviewing it, the psychoanalyst, Donald Winnicott,[162] argued that Jung's mother's mental illness when he was a child stopped her being alive to her own love and hate of Jung such that she never brought them imaginatively alive in him. Hence, wrote Winnicott, Jung's reliance on inanimate objects – the wooden manequin, for instance, which he made as a comforter for himself as a boy. Hence too his rooting the psyche in fixed complexes, symbols, and archetypes in the collective unconscious.

---

160 Hayman p. 426.

161 Hayman p. 122.

162 D. W. Winnicott (1964) Review of *Memories, Dreams, Reflections* by C. G. Jung, *IJPA*, **45** pp. 450–5.

Whether or not Jung's mother failed him by not bringing fully alive his capacity for love and hate, it seems Freud failed him by no sooner sensing his destructiveness than he made light of it in the case of Spielrein, and in the case of his destructiveness vis-à-vis psychoanalysis rejected him on this account. Without any affirmation of his destructiveness, according to Winnicott, Jung split it off and projected it into an image of God as evil as well as good. This might have contributed to Jung's empathy with, and pioneering work in extending psychoanalysis to understanding and treating the splitting occurring in schizophrenia. But it resulted, ultimately, in Jung misrepresenting both religion and psychoanalysis. As self-appointed apostle of therapy as means of revealing "the dark, subterranean God of each man's secret life", argued the sociologist, Philip Rieff, Jung developed a system that was true neither to religion nor to science.[163] Most of all, with his account of God as an archetype within us, Jung failed to address the outward- and other-directedness of religious experience. By contrast the political activist and theorist, Simone Weil, brought this out particularly well in her religious writings, as I will now seek to illustrate.

---

[163] P. Rieff (1966) *The Triumph of the Therapeutic: Uses of Faith after Freud*, London: Chatto & Windus.

Chapter 4

Simone Weil

Awaiting God

William James, as we have seen, described his father as belonging to

> that band of saints and mystics, whose [experience] . . . has always been an acute despair, passing over into an equally acute optimism, through a passion of self renunciation of the self and surrender to a higher power (see p. 19).

Simone Weil was just such a mystic. Her life also illustrates the excesses, as well as the virtues, of what William James called the fruits of saintliness – devotion, purity, and asceticism. Her life also indicates that religious or mystical experience may not be effective as therapy, at least for the headaches and anorexic self-starvation which she arguably psychosomatically inflicted on herself.

Nevertheless Weil's life also highlights the transformation to psychological life and health that William James described in terms of the literal and metaphorical illumination and light occurring both in religious conversion and in being in love. Her writing remains enormously inspiring in emphasizing the outward orientation of love to what is true and good as in the philosophy of Plato which, in her later life, she allied with Christian belief in God, as do others in their account of psychoanalysis and religion as I will explain in later chapters of this book. Accordingly this chapter will devote some space to Plato not least in relation to Simone Weil's early life.

Early philosophy

Plato recounts Socrates as arguing that knowledge of "absolute beauty, goodness, uprightness, holiness" precedes our birth. After that we can only know them indirectly through the reality available to us through our senses.[1] At the end of her life, Simone Weil, who had been an advocate of Plato's philosophy since her youth, similarly asserted: "There is a reality outside . . . man's mental

---

[1] Plato (n.d.) *Phaedo*, in *The Last Days of Socrates*, Harmondsworth: Penguin, pp. 97–183, 125.

universe . . . [which] is the source of all the good that can exist".[2] It is our capacity of directing "attention and love" to this reality "beyond the world and of receiving good from it", she said, that links and attaches us both to it and to our fellow human beings.[3] This other reality, beyond direct access to our bodily senses, is the locus, according to Plato, of what he called "the end of all endeavour, the object on which every heart is set". He called it "the Form of the Good".[4] Weil equated the good with God. "God is outside this world", she insisted. He is "the Good".[5] This is true and certain by definition. So too with faith. It consists, said Weil, in believing "that every thought of mine which is a desire for good brings me nearer to the good".[6]

Simone Weil wrote this in New York and London during her early 30s. Her life began, however, in Paris. She was born there on 3 February 1909 to Jewish parents. Like Jung's patient, Sabina Spielrein, Simone's mother was born in Rostov-on-Don, her father was born in Strasbourg. Simone was their second child.

Recalling her early life, Simone dated her first valuing attention to what is true and good to a period when she felt deeply depressed during her early teens at not being the mathematical genius her older brother, André, was already becoming. Or, as she put it:

> At fourteen I fell into one of those fits of bottomless despair which come with adolescence, and I seriously thought of dying because of the mediocrity of my natural faculties. The exceptional gifts of my brother, who had a childhood and youth comparable to those of Pascal, brought my own inferiority home to me. I did not mind having no visible successes, but what did grieve me was the idea of being excluded from that transcendent kingdom to which only the truly great have access and wherein truth abides. I preferred to die rather than live without that truth. After months of inward darkness, I suddenly had the everlasting conviction that no matter what human being, even though practically devoid of natural faculties, can penetrate to the kingdom of truth reserved for genius, if only he longs for truth and perpetually concentrates all his attention upon its attainment.[7]

It was, in a sense, a moment of secular conversion or transformation. Perhaps it contributed to her excellence as a student, recognized by her teacher,

---

[2] In M. D. Raper (1974) *Gateway to God*, Glasgow: Collins, p. 38.

[3] Ibid. p. 39.

[4] Plato (n.d.) *The Republic*, Harmondsworth: Penguin, 1955, pp. 169, 273.

[5] In Raper p. 41.

[6] Ibid. p. 43.

[7] Spiritual autobiography, 15 May 1942, in S. Weil (1950) *Waiting on God*, London: Fontana, pp. 18–49, 31.

Emile Chartier (also known as Alain), at the Lycée Henri IV, in assessing an essay she wrote for him, inspired by Plato's account of the insights he derived from poetry. The essay was about a story by the Brothers Grimm. It tells of a king who, to protect his six sons and daughter from his cruel wife, their step-mother, hides them in a forest. Finding the boys, however, the stepmother puts a magic silk shirt on each of them. The only way they can become human again, they tell their sister when she returns, is for her to sew for each of them a shirt from white anemones, as Weil put it, replacing the asters of the Grimms' story with white anemones to emphasize the delicacy and purity of the work to be done. She has to do it in six years without ever talking or laughing. So she begins and, despite her silence and seriousness, a king falls in love with her. They marry. But each time she has a baby the king's mother steals it and spreads rumours that her daughter-in-law has killed it. When this happens a third time the king reluctantly agrees to his wife being tried. Still staying silent, saying nothing in her defence, she is condemned to death whereupon, just as she is about to be executed, the six years now being nearly over, her brothers return. She throws the shirts she has made over them, and they become human again, all but her youngest brother who, because she has not quite fin-ished the second sleeve of his shirt, still has a wing in place of one of his arms. For Weil the point of the story, as one commentator puts it, is that:

> By attending to one thing only – the rescue of her brothers – the sister makes their existence and their humanity a solid reality, while the vicissitudes of everyday life in the royal household with the usual fears and hatreds and illusions of social life, dissip-ate it, as do the mysteries and dangers of the great forest.[8]

Weil likewise emphasized the importance of attending to oneness with others outside oneself in another essay for Alain, this time about Alexander the Great. She described how, parched with thirst when he and his men were crossing the desert, Alexander threw away water brought him from a long dis-tance away because, as Weil put it, were he to drink the water he would sep-arate himself from his men. "Everything takes place in Alexander's soul, and for him it is simply a matter of taking the stance of a man", commented Weil, "It is necessary therefore to save oneself, save the Spirit in oneself". It is a matter of refusing "to obey the animal in oneself".[9]

She devoted her graduating dissertation to the philosophy of Descartes. In it she emphasized that we are not only the passive object of reality, we also

---

[8] D. Avery (2002) Simone Weil's unfinished shirt, *PN Review*, **144** (March–April) pp. 28–33, 28.

[9] S. Pétrement (1976) *Simone Weil*, London: Mowbrays, p. 37.

actively engage with it. Describing this combination, she wrote:

> I am always two, on the one hand the passive being who submits to the world, on the other the active being who takes hold of it; geometry and physics make me conceive of how these two beings can be joined but do not join them. Can I not attain the perfect wisdom, wisdom in deed, which would join the two pieces of myself? I certainly cannot unite them directly because the presence of the world in my thoughts consists in this powerlessness; but I can unite them indirectly because action consists in nothing else. Not by that apparent action by which mad imagining makes me blindly overthrow the world of my chaotic desires, but real action, indirect action, action in accordance with geometry, or, to give it its true name, work.[10]

So saying, and despite the very severe headaches which she now began suffering, Weil did farm work as well as writing, teaching, and being a political activist. On graduating she combined secondary school teaching with workers' education classes aimed at enabling workers to know and understand the context and aim of their work. She was also involved, as a syndicalist, in union activity and wrote articles on the need to combine mental and manual labour rather than divide them as wrongly occurs, she said, in the managerialism of both Fascist and Marxist politics. She was nevertheless sympathetic with Marxism and even arranged for Trotsky to stay with her family at the end of 1933. In her major book, *Oppression and Liberty*, finished in autumn 1934, she emphasized the necessity to combine doing and thinking, movement and spirit. She described both as the essence of each worker's individuality and freedom from the tyranny of nature and society.

To get first hand experience of production line work she obtained employment in a factory in December 1934, and when this work ended, she got a job in another factory, and later, in 1935, worked as a milling machine operative for Renault. The work appalled her – the way it destroyed the spirit of both herself and her fellow-workers, making them unable to think or choose, by numbing and reducing them to senseless things, little better than the machines they operated. She described the alienation of her fellow-workers:

> One can actually see women waiting ten minutes outside a plant under a driving rain, across from an open door through which their bosses are passing. They are working women and they will not enter until the whistle has blown. That door is more alien to them than that of any strange house, which they would enter quite naturally if seeking cover.[11]

---

[10] S. Weil (1930) Introduction à science et perception dans Descartes, in S. Weil (1988) *Œuvres Complètes: I. Premiers écrits philosophiques*. Paris: Gallimard, p. 209.

[11] S. Weil (1943) Réflexions sur la vie d'usine, in G.A.Panichas (ed.) *The Simone Weil Reader*. New York: David McKay, 1977, pp. 53–72, 63.

She too became alienated from herself as a thing, devoid of all freedom and spirit.

> Here comes the foreman. "How many are you doing? 400 an hour? You need to do 800. Otherwise I can't keep you on. If you start doing 800 an hour from now on, I might consider keeping you". He talks without raising his voice. Why should he raise his voice when he can cause such anguish with one word? What to answer? "I'll try". Force the pace. Force it more. Every second overcome this paralyzing nausea, this disgust. Faster. Have to double the rhythm. How many have I done in this last hour? 650. The bell. Punch clock, change, go out of the factory, body drained of all its vital energy, spirit empty of thought, heart submerged in disgust, in dumb anger, and, overriding it all, a sense of impotence and submission. Because the only hope for the next day is that they might be willing to let me spend it in the same way.[12]

Herein lay the moment of "acute despair" akin to what William James' father called his Swedenborgian "vastation", and William called the source of "religious conversion" which, understood in Jungian terms, is a matter of symbolic transformation. For Simone Weil her healing transformation came through Christianity.

Christian transformation

Ill and defeated, Simone Weil left Renault soon after starting work there. On holiday with her parents in Portugal, she underwent the first of three transforming religious experiences. Going alone one evening to a desperately poor village when its inhabitants were celebrating the village's patron saint's day, she later recalled:

> The wives of the fishermen were going in procession to make a tour of all the ships, carrying candles and singing what must certainly be very ancient hymns of a heart-rending sadness. Nothing can give any idea of it. I have never heard anything so poignant unless it were the song of the boatmen on the Volga. There the conviction was suddenly borne in upon me that Christianity is pre-eminently the religion of slaves, that slaves cannot help belonging to it, and I among others.[13]

After more secondary school teaching, farm work, and briefly joining the anarchist militia in the Spanish civil war in July 1936 she had a second religious experience the next spring in Assisi:

> There, alone in the little twelfth-century Romanesque chapel of Santa Maria degli Angeli, an incomparable marvel of purity where Saint Francis often used to pray, something stronger than I was compelled me for the first time in my life to go down on my knees.[14]

....

[12] S. Weil (1936) La vie et la grève des ouvrières métallos, in S. Weil (1999) Œuvres, Paris: Gallimard, pp. 159–70, 160.

[13] In Weil 1950 pp. 33–4.

[14] Ibid. p. 34.

Again she did secondary school teaching. But her headaches were so bad she had to stop.

Her third transforming religious experience occurred the next Easter, 1938, when, going to Solesmes, and concentrating on "the unimaginable beauty of the chanting and the words" of the monks singing Gregorian chant in the monastery there, she said, "the thought of the Passion of Christ entered into my being once and for all".[15] Here, at Solesmes, she met an American, John Vernon, a student of English at Cambridge.[16] From him she gained what she called her "first idea of the supernatural power of the Sacraments because of the truly angelic radiance with which he seemed to be clothed after going to communion".[17]

Vernon introduced her to the work of the seventeenth century English metaphysical poets. She was particularly enchanted by a poem by the religious poet, George Herbert, which begins "Love bade me welcome: yet my soul drew back, / Guilty of dust and sin", and ends "You must sit down says Love, and taste my meat: / So I did sit and eat".[18] Concentrating all her attention on reciting this poem whenever her headaches were particularly bad, she began having mystical experiences. She wrote:

> Christ himself came down and took possession of me, neither my sense nor my imagination had any part; I only felt in the midst of my suffering the presence of a love, like that which one can read in the smile on a beloved face.[19]

This first occurred in November 1938. As well as being moved by Herbert's poem, *Love*, she was also moved by reading the Hindu *Bhagavad Gita* and Lao-Tse. They perfectly described, she wrote, the "waiting, attention, silence, immobility" of the passive activity of obedience.[20] The German occupation of Paris in June 1940 forced her and other Jews to become exiles. Together with her parents she left Paris and after some wandering settled in Marseilles. Here, in June 1941, she became involved in intense spiritual discussions with a blind Dominican priest, Joseph-Marie Perrin. Through him she also got work on a farm in the Ardèche run by a self-taught philosopher, Gustave Thibon, with whom she studied the Lord's Prayer in Greek. She now began reciting it every

---

[15] In Weil 1950 p. 34.

[16] Simone Weil herself recalled Vernon as English but according to the monks at Solesmes he was American.

[17] Weil 1950 p. 34.

[18] Ibid. p. 35 n.1.

[19] Ibid. pp. 35–6.

[20] Forms of the implicit love of God, in Weil 1950 pp. 94–166, 147.

morning with "absolutely pure attention".[21] It transported her to a mystical experience of oneness with a reality other than the finite world we ordinarily sense and perceive:

> At times the very first words tear my thoughts from my body and transport it to a place outside space where there is neither perspective nor point of view. The infinity of the ordinary expanses of perception is replaced by an infinity to the second or sometimes the third degree. At the same time, filling every part of this infinity of infinity, there is silence, a silence which is not an absence of sound but which is the object of a positive sensation, more positive than that of sound.[22]

She wrote more along these lines in a piece for Perrin about the importance of children enjoying their schoolwork because, she said, it develops their attention which, in being directed towards God, is the very substance of prayer. Attention depends on faith, she went on; its best support is love of God and knowing that if one asks Him for bread he will not give us a stone. Attention to what is beyond us is desire for light, for truth. It is attained through "suspending our thought, leaving it detached, empty and ready to be penetrated by the object".[23] Attention is not submission. It consists in watching and waiting. Its object is love of God and love of our neighbour recognized to be one with us. She also noted the contradiction involved in this oneness with the otherness of God.[24] In attention, she concluded her essay for Perrin, "the soul empties itself of all its own contents in order to receive into itself the being it is looking at, just as he is, in all his truth".[25] It involves consent. She likened it to a fiancée accepting her lover.[26]

In this and other essays written in the spring of 1942, and later collected together by Perrin in a book called *Attente de Dieu*, she also wrote about affliction. She wrote about it in religious terms and described the death of love that it can involve:

> Affliction makes God appear to be absent for a time, more absent than a dead man, more absent than light in the utter darkness of a cell. A kind of horror submerges the whole soul. During this absence there is nothing to love. What is terrible is that if, in

[21] Ibid. p. 38.

[22] Ibid.

[23] Reflections on the right use of school studies with a view to the love of God, April 1942, in Weil 1950 pp. 66–76, 72.

[24] "*C'est que nous sommes contradiction, étant des créatures, étant Dieu et infiniment autres que Dieu.*" S. Weil (1942) *Œuvres Complètes tome VI: Cahiers 8–12 [February to July 1942], La porte du transcendant*, Paris: Gallimard, 2002, p. 96.

[25] Weil 1950 p. 75.

[26] Ibid. p. 146.

this darkness, there is nothing to love, the soul ceases to love, God's absence becomes final.[27]

The answer lies in nevertheless continuing loving. The soul, she said, "has to go on loving in the emptiness, or at least to go on wanting to love, though it may only be with an infinitesimal part of itself".[28] She likened it to the immeasurable point, except in so far as it is visually represented, where a tangent touches a circle, designating the place where two different entities meet.[29] In her essay on affliction she went on "if the soul stops loving it falls, even in this life, into something which is almost equivalent to hell".[30] But, she maintained,

> The greatest suffering, so long as it does not cause fainting, does not touch the part of the soul which consents to right direction. It is only necessary to know that love is a direction and not a state of the soul. If one is unaware of this, one falls into despair at the first onslaught of affliction.[31]

Keeping one's attention directed towards God centres one at the very heart of life. Or so she said.

Confronted with affliction what are we to do? The answer, Weil indicated, lies in discovering in the afflicted their capacity for freedom and consent. Awakening their freedom – their spirit – involves becoming one with them. Or, as Weil put it, "To wish for the existence of this free consent in another, deprived of it by affliction, is to transport oneself into him".[32] It entails love – "Love sees what is invisible". Putting this in religious terms, she added that only God has "the power really to think into being that which does not exist".[33] It is through Him, but we could also say in non-religious terms that it is through love, through being oriented by and wanting to love, that we find the life and light of the spirit threatened with obliteration in affliction. Weil expressed this, and the obstacles to realizing love, again in terms of God:

> Difficult as it is really to listen to someone in affliction, it is just as difficult for him to know that compassion is listening to him. The love of our neighbour is love which comes down from God to man . . . though it finds no name for him, wherever the afflicted are loved for themselves alone, it is God who is present.[34]

---

[27] Weil 1950 p. 80.

[28] Ibid. p. 80.

[29] Weil 1942 p. 258.

[30] Weil 1950 p. 80.

[31] Ibid. p. 93.

[32] Ibid. p. 104.

[33] Ibid. p. 106.

[34] Ibid. pp. 106, 107.

This, she wrote, entails "attention to the victim of affliction as to a being and not a thing; it means wishing to preserve in him the faculty of free consent".[35] It entails attending to the other not as object of need but as their own centre of freedom, love, choice, and consent. What is good and needed may coexist. But, warns Weil, "When the attachment of one being to another is made up of need and nothing else it is a fearful thing". For, she argued,

> When a human being is attached to another by a bond of affection which contains any degree of necessity, it is impossible that he should wish autonomy to be preserved both in himself and in the other.[36]

The answer lies not in need and pity but in love of one's neighbour as having the same separateness and autonomy as oneself. Reaffirming this Christian doctrine, Weil also described in religious and mathematical terms the resolution of the oneness with, and separation from others involved:

> It is impossible for two human beings to be one while scrupulously respecting the distance which separates them, unless God is present in each of them. The point at which parallels meet is infinity.[37]

Loving another in their oneness with, and freedom from us is no easy matter especially when they are afflicted, as of course those seeking therapy often are. In notes Weil gave Thibon, which he collected together into a book, published in English as *Gravity and Grace*, Weil criticized Freudian therapy:

> All the Freudian system is impregnated with the prejudice which it makes it its mission to fight – the prejudice that everything sexual is vile. There is an essential difference between the mysticism which turns towards God the faculty of love and desire of which sexual energy constitutes the physiological foundation, and the false imitation of mysticism which, without changing the natural orientation of this faculty, gives it an imaginary object upon which it stamps the name of God as a label. To discriminate between these two operations, of which the second is still lower than debauchery, is difficult, but it is possible.[38]

True mysticism, she indicated, involves recognizing that "God and the supernatural are hidden and formless in the universe".[39] They are not to be captured in imaginary objects and labels. God exists outside our world of words and things.

She advocated emptying oneself of all imagined and remembered objects from the future and past, bearing with the emptiness so as to make way for God.

---

[35] Ibid. p. 109.

[36] Ibid. pp. 155, 156.

[37] Ibid. p. 160.

[38] S. Weil (1947) *Gravity and Grace*, London: Routledge, 1952, p. 49.

[39] Ibid. p. 49.

Or, as she put it,

> He enters into contact with a human individual as such only through purely spiritual grace which responds to the gaze turned towards him, that is to say to the exact extent to which the individual ceases to be an individual.[40]

Opening oneself, through attention, to God understood as outside oneself – not one with the self as in Jung's version of therapy – does not entail exerting one's will. It is not achieved through gritting one's teeth, tensing one's muscles, or setting one's jaw "about virtue, or poetry, or the solution of a problem".[41] Rather, attention is a matter of faith in, and love of what is good. "If we turn our mind toward the good", Weil maintained, "it is impossible that little by little the whole soul will not be attracted thereto in spite of itself".[42] It is not a matter of will. It is a matter of "desire – or more exactly, consent".[43] Full attention to the object brings truth and goodness. The perception of beauty comes from simply desiring that the object on which one fixes one's attention should exist. It unites the instantaneous and eternal. Putting Plato's theory of forms in theistic terms, Weil emphasized that beauty is "an incarnation of God in the world".[44]

After giving her notes about this to Thibon, Weil left Marseilles on 14 May 1942 for New York, where her brother was living with his family. A couple of days before leaving Marseilles she wrote to a friend, Joë Bousquet, about her experience of affliction, her headaches:

> A moment came when I thought I was threatened, by exhaustion and deepening pain, with such a hideous downfall of my whole soul, that for several weeks I wondered with anguish if to die was not the most pressing duty, though it seemed appalling that my life should end in horror. As I told you, only a resolution of conditional and timely death restored me to serenity.[45]

On the journey to New York, while staying in a transit camp in Casablanca, she wrote about oneness with the affliction of others and how it can almost obliterate one's sense of love or of God:

> When I am in contact with the affliction of other people ... contact causes me such atrocious pain and so utterly rends my soul, that as a result the love of God becomes almost impossible for me for a while.[46]

---

[40] S. Weil (1947) *Gravity and Grace*, London: Routledge, 1952, p. 101.

[41] Ibid. p. 105.

[42] Ibid. p. 106.

[43] Ibid. p. 107.

[44] Ibid. p. 137.

[45] To Joë Bousquet, 12 May 1942, in Weil 1999 pp. 793–800, 797.

[46] To Perrin from Casablanca, 26 May 1942, in Weil 1950 p. 55.

Brought up in "complete agnosticism", she went on, she had nevertheless become delivered into "Christ's hand" by "the beauty of the world".[47] But for this self-same reason she refused to join the Catholic church because of the harm it can do to the truth and to others – as it had in the inquisition and as it continued to do through its nationalism in Catholic countries.

Soon after arriving in New York she left, that November, for London, where she worked with the Free French on plans for France's post-war regeneration. In this connection she wrote a book, *The Need for Roots*. In it she again dwelt on the direction given attention by love of others outside us. She compared a pregnant woman sewing a layette, mindful of her love for her baby growing inside her, with a woman in prison, compelled by fear to sew well lest she get punished. What is needed, wrote Weil, is a society which enables everyone to work like the first woman, with love and knowledge of why and what they are doing.

Weil also dwelt in *The Need for Roots* on mysticism. In mystics, she marvelled, truth becomes life. The same happens in science. Properly practised it too has a direction. Its object is truth and love. To highlight the point she compared a man who discovers that the wife he loves is unfaithful to him with a man who learns that someone he does not know has been unfaithful to her husband. The former alone, wrote Weil, involves truth, because it involves love. "Pure and genuine love", she went on, "always desires above all to dwell wholly in the truth whatever it may be, unconditionally . . . It is the Holy Spirit".[48] The "spirit of truth", she maintained, only dwells in science provided the scientist is motivated by "love of the object which forms the stuff of his investigations". The scientist's true aim, she added, is "the union of his own mind with the mysterious wisdom eternally inscribed in the universe". She accordingly called scientific investigation "a form of religious contemplation".[49] As for the regeneration of France, she concluded that its "spiritual core" should be centred on work based not on coercion but on freely directed choice and consent.[50]

She herself now became very ill whilst working in London. In April 1943 she was hospitalized with TB and might have recovered had she eaten more. Out of fellow-feeling with those with whom she had worked in Paris, then deprived of food by the German occupation, she ate very little. She became very weak and was sent from London to a sanatorium in Ashford in Kent where a few

---

47 Ibid. p. 58.

48 S. Weil (1949) *The Need for Roots*, London: Routledge & Kegan Paul, 1952, p. 242.

49 Ibid. p. 250.

50 Ibid. p. 287.

days later she died, on 24 August 1943. "French Professor starves herself to death", reported one local newspaper. Another announced more respectfully, "French Professor's curious sacrifice".[51] In 1951 the Algerian novelist, Albert Camus, declared her "*le seul grande esprit de notre temps*".[52] Over half a century later the Cambridge theologian, Donald Cupitt, noted how Simone Weil had inspired Iris Murdoch to abandon what he called the "masculinism" of the will for novels celebrating "the cultivation of the contemplative values".[53] The same year the French novelist and critic, Philippe Sollers, welcomed the publication of another volume of her notebooks, *La Porte du Transcendant*.[54]

Simone Weil was a mystic, not a therapist. Nevertheless she arguably turned Christian Platonism to therapeutic effect in recovering, through it, from the despairing self-alienation and numbness she suffered in factory work during the mid-1930s. Becoming a Christian Platonist entailed adopting a quite different version of truth from that of William James. Whereas he regarded truth, pragmatically, as what works, Weil regarded truth and goodness as inhering in God as ultimate being, outside and beyond us, inspiring our attention, love, and life. Towards the end of her life she wrote of goodness and God:

> Outside me there is a good which is superior to me and which influences me for good every time that I desire the good. Since there is no possible limit to this operation, this external good is infinite, it is God.[55]

Sadly this philosophy of the superiority of God and goodness went hand in hand for Weil with self-hating anti-semitism, and sometimes repulsively self-punishing masochism. In the quote with which I began this chapter, William James talked of the therapeutic effects of religious conversion or transformation in terms of "self renunciation . . . to a higher power". Such renunciation risks not only masochism but also authoritarianism, as I will explain in turning to Erich Fromm's approach to psychoanalysis and religion.

---

[51] In D. McLellan (1990) *Utopian Pessimist*, New York: Poseidon Press, p. 266.

[52] In P. Sollers (2002) Resistance de Simone Weil, *Le Monde de Livres*, 26 April, p. 1.

[53] D. Cupitt (2002) Iris and the death of God, *The Guardian*, 23 March, p. 20.

[54] P. Sollers (2002) Resistance de Simone Weil, *Le Monde de Livres*, 26 April, p. 1.

[55] In Raper p. 41.

Chapter 5

Erich Fromm

Humanist Buddhism

Simone Weil wrote very much as a woman. She was not a feminist and indeed was so unsympathetic to feminism that she gave her workers' education classes on the subject to someone else to teach. Nevertheless her account of waiting on, and attending to, God is suffused with imagery of a woman awaiting her lover in sex.

The sociologist and psychoanalyst, Erich Fromm, by contrast, paid scant attention to love, sex, or women. Instead he cast what he had to say about psychoanalysis and religion in terms of individual men freeing themselves to realize their power and potential. His male-centredness and rampant individualism is off-putting. Yet, cast in more gender-neutral terms, his plea for humanistic religion, Buddhism, and psychoanalysis as means of enabling us to recover oneness with the world is appealing. His plea for us to become free from alienating our responsibility for choosing and doing into others idealized or deified as superego gods within or outside us is also a welcome antidote to the masochistic self-surrender of religious and mystical experience all too often evident in Simone Weil's life and work. To highlight this I will begin with Fromm's early anti-authoritarianism.

Anti-authoritarianism

Erich Fromm was born in Protestant-dominated Frankfurt on 23 March 1900 into an ethnic minority, a Jewish family. True to his family's name ("Fromm" means "pious") he studied the Old Testament as a boy. He also became interested in psychology, he said, because of his own and his parents' neuroses and because of the suicide of a 25-year-old painter friend of the family when Fromm was 12. The hysterical xenophobic propaganda of the First World War also made him interested in psychoanalysis and in social psychology. After the war, and after completing his doctoral dissertation (about the social psychology of three Jewish communities), he edited a small Jewish newspaper. In 1924 he abandoned his previous ambition to become a rabbi and decided to become a psychoanalyst. He went into analysis with Frieda Reichmann, whom he soon after married, and with whom he founded, together with others, an institute of psychoanalysis. Later he also joined the Frankfurt Institute of Social Research, and wrote a number of articles about social psychology, religion and psychoanalysis.

Following Hitler's rise to power in 1933 he left Frankfurt for Geneva and then went to New York where he arrived at the end of May 1934. Here, now separated from Frieda Reichmann, he continued working as a sociologist and psychoanalyst, and wrote articles for the US journal, *Psychiatry*, which formed the basis of one of his best known books, *Fear of Freedom* (also known as *Escape from Freedom*).

Published in 1941, Fromm's central aim in this book was to understand, in psychoanalytic terms, the historical and religious determinants of the authoritarianism of Hitler's Germany. In doing so Fromm revised Freud's instinct theory into a psychological theory more attuned to the historically changing social factors shaping human psychology. Beginning with the communal fellow-feeling between people of feudalism, Fromm described how this was overthrown by capitalism freeing people to sell their labour power as individuals on their own account.

But this freedom was achieved at a cost. Individuals found themselves "left alone", without the security of their previous "traditional status" and sense of "belonging".[1] Hence the appeal, wrote Fromm, of Martin Luther, in the early sixteenth century. In challenging and freeing his followers from the authority of the medieval church, explained Fromm, Luther quelled their fear of freedom and of doubt with the certainty of a creed preaching that human beings are innately evil and can only achieve God's grace through humiliating and demolishing their "individual will and pride".[2] Luther thereby freed people from one authority only to submit them to another, to "a God who insisted on complete submission of man and annihilation of the individual self as the essential condition to his salvation".[3] This in turn made people ready to alienate themselves as objects to be used by others for economic productivity and capital accumulation.

Calvin similarly taught people to allay their fear of freedom through the security of self-submission to God. Calvin's doctrine of predestination, furthermore, taught people that they are basically unequal. In doing so it undermined solidarity between them. Moreover, Calvinism emphasized that people

---

[1] E. Fromm (1941) *Escape from Freedom*, New York: Avon Books, 1965 pp. 77, 80.

[2] Ibid. p. 94.

[3] Ibid. p. 100.

should submit to an internal master relentlessly driving them to succeed in work without ever allowing them to enjoy themselves: "Success became the sign of God's grace; failure, the sign of damnation".[4] Psychoanalysing this position, Fromm contended that in submitting to Calvin's "despotic God"[5] people repressed their resulting hostility and resentment, and projected it onto others or turned it against themselves.

This situation was exacerbated in Germany by its defeat in the First World War, by the decimation of its pre-war empire, by the growing power of monopolies, and by post-war inflation. All this contributed to the willingness of the German lower middle class to submit to the authoritarianism of Nazi ideology and to Hitler as their leader. The rise of Nazism could be understood in terms of Freud's theory of the internalized authority of the superego. Internalizing or projecting this authority onto others is a means of escaping freedom, choice, doubt, and responsibility for oneself. Or we avoid freedom, independence, and separation from others through masochistically depending on them as objects of our sadistic control. Hence the sado-masochism of the authoritarian personality.

Fromm did not agree with Freud that it is sex that needs to be freed; rather what needs freeing is what Fromm called "the spontaneous activity of the total integrated personality".[6] Individuals might have abrogated their freedom in the name of Lutheran or Calvinist Protestantism, or in the name of German Fascism, but psychoanalysis – focusing not on biological or sexual instinct but on the individuality of the self – could help free us: "psychological forces", concluded Fromm, "are molded by the external conditions of life, but they also have a dynamism of their own".[7]

Fromm's voluntaristic conclusion that we can, by implication, free ourselves from authoritarianism by exerting our will against it, reiterated his book's initial proclamation; namely, that the answer to authoritarianism in politics and religion lies in a revised version of Freudian psychoanalysis affirming people's capacity to act on, rather than evade the individual freedom won for them by capitalism. With this celebration of what is a fundamental tenet of US individualism, Fromm's book became a best-seller.

With its publication Fromm began teaching at the New School of Social Research in New York where he also ran seminars with the German-born

---

4 Ibid. p. 112.

5 Ibid. p. 116.

6 Ibid. p. 284.

7 Ibid. p. 326.

theologian, Paul Tillich, on psychoanalysis and religion. He also wrote about what he called rational and irrational religious and secular belief. Belief is irrational, he said, if it is an effect of submission to others because of their power rather than because of any skill or ability they might have. As illustration Fromm cited the Jews who, on being liberated from Egypt by Moses, continued to want to submit to God as someone who proved His power through miracles and magic rather than believe in Him, as God wanted, on the basis of their own experience. Rational belief, by contrast, arises spontaneously, said Fromm, from "genuine intellectual and emotional activity".[8]

Fromm reiterated this argument in his next book, *Man for Himself*. In it he commended Freud's passionate commitment to the truth. But he rejected Freud's later account of health in terms of shoring up the defences of the ego, or at least the defence of the superego as an inner figure of authority. Health, explained Fromm, does not consist in submitting to the superego, to God, nor to any other authority. It consists in self-realization. Putting this in religious terms, Fromm approvingly quoted the Christian mystic, Meister Eckhart:

> That I am a man, this I share with other men. That I see and hear and that I eat and drink is what all animals do likewise. But that I am I is only mine and belongs to me and to nobody else; to no other man nor to an angel nor to God – except inasmuch as I am one with Him.[9]

Fromm further developed his anti-authoritarian emphasis on people recovering their freedom to realize themselves as individuals when he gave the Terry Lectures at Yale in 1949.

Humanism

Fromm's Terry Lectures were published the next year as a book, *Psychoanalysis and Religion*. In it he countered what he called the authoritarianism of Jung's religious version of psychoanalysis with what he called the humanism of Freud's theory. Jung's authoritarianism is evident, Fromm wrote, in his characterizing religious experience in terms of surrendering to a higher power – God – in the unconscious. In this Jung's account of religious experience is akin to that of those escaping feelings of aloneness and limitation through submission to Calvinism. In Jung's system, as well as in authoritarian religion, claimed Fromm, people can only discover themselves indirectly through God. Furthermore, in believing in God in this fashion, they project what is best of themselves into God. The believer thereby empties himself, thus adding to his

---

[8] E. Fromm (1942) Faith as a character trait, *Psychiatry* 5 pp. 307–19, 313.

[9] E. Fromm (1947) *Man for Himself*, New York: Holt, Rinehart & Winston, p. 38.

self-alienation: "The emptier he becomes, the more sinful he feels. The more sinful he feels, the more he praises his God – and the less able he is to regain himself".[10]

Humanism, by contrast, involves recognizing and realizing our freedom as individuals. Fromm approved, in these terms, Freud's argument that, as Fromm put it, we must free ourselves from the infantile illusion of a fatherly God, and instead develop and make use of the capacities within us which are the only powers on which we can rely. Humanism, Fromm contended, lies at the heart of what is best in the religious teaching of the Buddha, Lao-Tse, the Prophets, and Jesus. Humanism centres on man developing "his power of reason in order to understand himself, his relationship to his fellow men and his position in the universe".[11] Humanistic religious experience, Fromm went on, is "experience of oneness with the All . . . grasped with thought and with love".[12] In so far as humanistic religions are theistic, God in such religions "is a symbol of *man's own powers* which he tries to realize in his life".[13] Reiterating the point, Fromm wrote "in humanistic religion God is the image of man's higher self, a symbol of what man potentially is or ought to become", rather than a projection of what is best in him into someone else, as in Jung's authoritarian, psychoanalytic version of religious experience in terms of an archetype of God in the collective unconscious.

The true psychoanalytic "physician of the soul", wrote Fromm – adopting from Plato this epithet as did Freud's friend, Pfister – seeks to achieve the "optimal development of a person's potentialities and the realization of his individuality . . . independence, integrity, and the ability to love".[14] In both humanistic religion and psychoanalysis the search for the truth is held to be inseparably linked to attaining freedom and independence. Translating Freud's theory of incest and the Oedipus complex into ego or self psychology, Fromm argued that incest is another name for our longing to remain attached to our parents rather than experience ourselves as separate and responsible for what we do.

Just as Freud advocated freeing ourselves from primary narcissistic oneness with, and dependence on our parents to face reality on our own account, argued Fromm, so do all great religions. The Buddha, for instance, demanded

---

[10] E. Fromm (1950) *Psychoanalysis and Religion*, New Haven: Yale University Press, p. 51.

[11] Ibid. p. 37.

[12] Ibid. p. 37.

[13] Ibid. p. 37.

[14] Ibid. p. 74.

that people should rid themselves of "familiar" ties to find strength in themselves.[15] The psychoanalytic cure of the soul aims to help patients likewise "to gain the faculty to see the truth, to love, to become free and responsible".[16] Psychoanalysis thereby promotes the following, threefold humanistic religious experience:

> [1] the wondering, the marveling, the becoming aware of life and of one's own existence, and of the puzzling problem of one's relatedness to the world . . . [2] what Paul Tillich has called the "ultimate concern" . . . with the meaning of life, with the self-realization of man, with the fulfillment of the task which life sets us . . . [3] oneness not only in oneself, not only with one's fellow men, but with all life and, beyond that, with the universe.[17]

In the same year as Fromm's Terry lectures were published, he moved to Mexico with his second wife, Henny (whom he had married in 1944), in the hope that its climate might be good for her health. But she died soon after and Fromm remarried in 1953. He stayed in Mexico and became director of a department of psychoanalysis in one of its university medical schools. He also continued writing about religion and psychoanalysis. He now advocated what he called "Humanistic Communitarian Socialism".[18] Through redistributing property, he envisaged, humanistic socialism would create a sane society in which, instead of deadening and self-alienating conformity with others, people might realize their individual potential through love and work.

Many were critical of Fromm's recipe for a sane society. Paul Tillich, whom he had cited favourably in his Terry lectures, criticized his book in religious terms. He asked:

> Is not the self-loss of man in the present society a consequence of the loss of God in the preceding period? Is true humanism possible without a consciousness of something that transcends man? . . . How can alienated man overcome alienation by himself?[19]

In a sense Fromm answered Tillich's questions in his next book, *The Art of Loving*. In it he emphasized not individual self-love but love of others as antidote to our tendency to take flight from freedom in self-alienating submission to the authority of, and conformity with, others. He linked love with the

[15] E. Fromm (1950) *Psychoanalysis and Religion*, New Haven: Yale University Press, p. 84.

[16] Ibid. p. 92.

[17] Ibid. pp. 94–5.

[18] E. Fromm (1955) *The Sane Society*, London: Routledge, 1963 p. 363.

[19] P. Tillich (1955) Erich Fromm's "The Sane Society", *Pastoral Psychology* (September) pp. 13–6, 16.

transcendence of what he now called "mature" religion in contrast to love of God based on immature, infantile love of one's parents. Mature religion, he wrote, involves recognizing our limitations, our not knowing anything about God, for instance. Love of God in Western religion consists not of knowledge but of intellectual belief in His existence, justice, and love. In mysticism and Eastern religion, by contrast, love of God consists of an intense emotional "feeling experience of oneness, inseparably linked with the expression of this love in every act of living".[20]

Zen Buddhism

In August 1957 Fromm moved to Cuernavaca, where he helped run a workshop devoted to Zen Buddhism and psychoanalysis. The book resulting from this workshop begins with an essay by the Zen Buddhist, Suzuki. It continues with an essay by Fromm in which he points out that whilst psychoanalysis is a form of therapy, Zen Buddhism is "a way to spiritual salvation".[21] Psychoanalysis, he went on, emerged out of the split since Descartes in the western psyche between reason and emotion, with the former so dominating and controlling nature in the production of things that human existence likewise became dominated by having rather than being. Religion declined, and Nietzsche famously declared that God was dead.

The notion of God as a fatherly helper was abandoned. So too were "the true aims of all great humanistic religions",[22] namely, according to Fromm, that of becoming what one potentially is. In seeking to achieve this aim, he argued, psychoanalysis and Zen Buddhism are alike. Their similarities include their both believing that knowing oneself transforms one, the attempt by psychoanalysis to deconstruct through free association the west's usually highly valued conscious thinking, and its not limiting this process in terms of time or money.

Defining health, as does today's World Health Organization, not as "absence of illness" but as "presence of well-being",[23] Fromm equated the latter with being aware of ourselves as separate beings in "oneness with the world".[24] This entails, he said, not regressing to the state of unity of ourselves as babies with

---

[20] E. Fromm (1956) *The Art of Loving*, London: Allen & Unwin, 1957 p. 80.

[21] E. Fromm (1960) Psychoanalysis and Zen Buddhism, in D. T. Suzuki, E. Fromm and R. de Martino (1960) *Zen Buddhism and Psychoanalysis*, London: Allen & Unwin, p. 77.

[22] Ibid. p. 80.

[23] Ibid. p. 86.

[24] Ibid. p. 87.

our mothers or fathers before we were ever aware of reality outside us. It entails not regressing to what Fromm called "prehuman, preconscious . . . animal" existence.[25] It entails being "fully awake . . . emerging fully from prehuman existence, by developing the specifically human potentiality of reason and love".[26]

Recovering our well-being entails not regressing to the unity of primary narcissism described by Freud in his 1927 book about religion, *The Future of an Illusion*. Rather it involves arriving at a "new unity . . . in which reason no longer separates man from his immediate, intuitive grasp of reality".[27] Its goal is variously symbolized as "Tao, Nirvana, Enlightenment, the Good, God".[28] Both Judaeo-Christian and Buddhist thinking argue that transforming enlightenment entails giving up one's "will".[29] In Zen terminology this is often called making oneself empty. Better this, suggested Fromm, than the Christian terminology of emptying oneself to God with its implication that one thereby alienates responsibility for one's "decisions into an omniscient, omnipotent father".[30]

Fromm then turned to what he claimed was Freud's psychoanalytic version of what Zen Buddhism calls enlightenment, namely becoming conscious of what was unconscious. Freud discovered, Fromm noted, that this entails not merely acquiring intellectual knowledge through, for instance, the analyst's interpretations or not merely knowing something about oneself as a separate object. Rather it entails experiencing this object of knowledge from within. The experience is transforming. "One's eyes are suddenly opened", wrote Fromm.[31] At first it is anxiety-making and then, like a mystical Swedenborgian "vastation", as William James' father might have put it, insight is followed by a sense of seeing the light. It is succeeded by what Fromm called "a new feeling of strength and certainty".[32]

In its account of the transforming character of becoming conscious of what was unconscious, wrote Fromm, psychoanalysis went beyond the usual subject–object split of western knowing. But Freud wrongly overlooked the fact that this depends on the analyst also abandoning western philosophy's

[25] E. Fromm (1960) Psychoanalysis and Zen Buddhism, in D. T. Suzuki, E. Fromm and R. de Martino (1960) *Zen Buddhism and Psychoanalysis*, London: Allen & Unwin, p. 93.

[26] Ibid. pp. 91, 93–4.

[27] Ibid. p. 94.

[28] Ibid. p. 94.

[29] Ibid. p. 94.

[30] Ibid. p. 95.

[31] Ibid. p. 110.

[32] Ibid. p. 110.

usual subject–object split in relating to his patient. Psychoanalysts, said Fromm, should abandon this detached, interpretative stance, as Freud's follower, Ferenczi, recognized in advocating that the analyst should love the patient with the love the patient needed but did not experience as a child. This entails the analyst experiencing in himself what the patient experiences. It entails the analyst "being soaked with the patient".[33] This in turn depends on the analyst overcoming "his own alienation and separateness".[34]

In this, Fromm went on, the analyst becomes like the master in Zen Buddhism, the essence of whose aim is "acquisition of enlightenment (*satori*) . . . the art of seeing into the nature of one's being . . . the full awakening of the personality to reality".[35] This entails not being blinded by greed, fear, wishing, or fantasizing. Enlightenment is "complete aliveness", intense experience of the object from within as what it is in itself, or, as Fromm also put it, "I bring it to life – and it brings me to life".[36] *Satori*, wrote Fromm, is akin to Plato's story of men leaving a cave, in which they mistake shadows for reality, going into the light and seeing reality itself. More than this, Zen aims at non-alienated self-knowledge "in which knower and known become one".[37]

The psychoanalyst is not a teacher, nor is the Zen master. He is a Zen master only in so far as he conveys "the only thing that can be conveyed: his existence".[38] He is, as it were, a "midwife" –[39] a catalyst. Similarly the analyst's responsibility resides, said Fromm, in "giving himself to the patient in search of the aim the patient seeks him for".[40] Zen Buddhist enlightenment, becoming conscious of what was unconscious, entails returning to the "undistorted grasp of reality" of the child after having gone through the subsequent stage of the subject–object split of knowing oneself and others. With enlightenment one is again in tune with reality: "I am open to it; I let it be".[41] Spinoza, said Fromm, called this form of knowing "intuition".[42]

---

[33] Ibid. p. 112.

[34] Ibid. p. 113.

[35] Ibid. pp. 114–16.

[36] Ibid. p. 117.

[37] Ibid. p. 118.

[38] Ibid. p. 120.

[39] Ibid. p. 125.

[40] Ibid. p. 126.

[41] Ibid. p. 130.

[42] Ibid. p. 133.

In seeking what Zen Buddhism calls enlightenment, psychoanalysis is not just a matter of treating symptoms. Its aim is not absence of illness. Rather its aim is the well-being of the oneness of "immediate and uncontaminated grasp of the world".[43] Its aim is not "reform" but "transformation" through analysts experiencing "oneness" with their patients.[44] Just as Suzuki said that one candle brings light into a dark room, with further candles increasing the light, so each insight in analysis "opens a door", as Fromm put it, to the patient no longer closing himself off from "being and becoming himself".[45]

Fromm's essay to this effect was published in 1960. He remained in Cuernavaca until 1974 when he moved with his wife to Switzerland, where he continued writing about religion and psychoanalysis. His last book was about Freud. It was published in 1979.[46] Having suffered several heart attacks, he died the following year, on 18 March 1980, leaving a body of work which remains a major inspiration of current writing about psychoanalysis and religion, to which I will return later in this book. More immediately I will now consider the existentialist theology of Paul Tillich.

---

[43] E. Fromm (1960) Psychoanalysis and Zen Buddhism, in D. T. Suzuki, E. Fromm and R. de Martino (1960) *Zen Buddhism and Psychoanalysis*, London: Allen & Unwin, p. 136.

[44] Ibid. pp. 136, 138.

[45] Ibid. p. 139.

[46] E. Fromm (1979) *Sigmund Freuds Psychoanalyse – Grösse und Grenzen*, Stuttgart: Deutsche Verlags-Anstalt.

Chapter 6

Paul Tillich

Being accepted

Paul Tillich is not immediately appealing. Within feminist theology he has been pilloried because of revelations after his death by his widow about his sexual proclivities.[1] Furthermore, in subscribing to Protestant belief in God, Tillich's writings about religion and psychoanalysis are not readily appealing to non-Protestant Christians, to members of other religions, nor to those of us who have no belief in God.

Nevertheless his work is also attractive. It is a welcome antidote to those who, like Erich Fromm, combine religion and psychoanalysis through turning both into recipes for self-sufficient individualism. It is also a welcome antidote to Jung's belief in the psyche surviving death in so far as he credited spiritualism and argued for the existence of an inherited collective unconscious. Tillich, by contrast, in espousing existentialism, insisted on our not surviving after death. He insisted on the fact of our mortality, on the fact of our nothingness before and after life. This does not sound very attractive. But what he insists on is also true. What is also appealing, at least in my view, is his attention, like that of William James, to personal experience, and his insistence on the intersubjective character of healing self-division through accepting being accepted, as I will explain later in this chapter, after beginning with his childhood and youth.

Early experience

Consistent with his existentialist philosophy which emphasizes the limits of human existence, Tillich later recorded that, when he was first born, on 20 August 1886 (in a small East German town, Startzeddel, near Berlin), he was so frail it seemed his existence might be very short-lived. His baptism, by his Lutheran pastor father, Johannes, was accordingly postponed. But Paul survived. So too did his two younger sisters, Johanna and Elisabeth and in the

---

[1] H. Tillich (1973) *From Time to Time*, New York: Stein & Day; and M. Daly (1978) *Gyn/Ecology*, London: The Women's Press, pp. 94–5.

early 1890s the family moved to Schönfliess-Neumark where Johannes became superintendent of the diocese there. Paul later wrote that it was here that he first experienced what he called "an indestructible good".[2] Or, as he also put it:

> My love for church buildings and their mystic atmosphere, for liturgy and music and sermons, and for the great Christian festivals that molded the life of the town for days and even weeks of the year left an indelible feeling in me for the ecclesiastical and sacramental. To these must be added the mysteries of Christian doctrine and their impact on the inner life of a child, the language of the Scriptures, and the exciting experiences of holiness, guilt, and forgiveness.[3]

He was also early moved by "the idea of the Infinite"[4] conveyed by the mystery of land and sea:

> Nearly all the great memories and longings of my life are interwoven with landscapes, soil, weather, the fields of grain and the smell of the potato plant in autumn, the shapes of clouds, and with wind, flowers and woods . . . . The weeks and, later, months that I spent by the sea every year from the time I was eight were even more important for my life and work. The experience of the infinite bordering on the finite suited my inclination toward the boundary situation and supplied my imagination with a symbol that gave substance to my emotions and creativity to my thought . . . . The sea also supplied the imaginative element necessary for the doctrines of the Absolute as both ground and abyss of dynamic truth, and of the substance of religion as the thrust of the eternal into finitude.[5]

When he was 12 he was sent to secondary school in Königsberg, where he allayed the loneliness of boarding away from home by reading the Bible. With his father's move to a post in Berlin, however, he went to school there, beginning in early 1901, and the next year he was confirmed by his father for which he chose the text "Come unto me all ye that labour and are heavy laden",[6] complementing his father's chosen text, "The truth will set you free".[7] Feeling heavy laden himself through his mid-teens, he later wrote that he often withdrew into Shakespeare and into other "imaginary worlds which seemed to be truer than the world outside".[8] Then, when he was just 17, his mother died from cancer. She was only 43.

---

[2] P. Tillich (1964) Autobiographical reflections, in C. W. Kegley and R. W. Bretall (eds) *The Theology of Paul Tillich*, New York: Macmillan, pp. 3–21, 6.

[3] P. Tillich (1936) *On the Boundary: An autobiographical sketch*, London: Collins, 1967, p. 59.

[4] Ibid. p. 30.

[5] Ibid. pp. 17, 18.

[6] P. Tillich (1949) The yoke of religion, in *The Shaking of the Foundations*, Harmondsworth: Penguin, 1962, pp. 99–108, 99.

[7] In W. Pauck and M. Pauck (1977) *Paul Tillich: His Life and Thought*, London: Collins, p. 13.

[8] Tillich 1936 p. 24.

Perhaps the shortness of her existence contributed, in part, to his now pursuing the philosophies of existence of Schelling and Kierkegaard at various universities – in Berlin, Tübingen, Halle, and Breslau – at which he then studied. From 1906 to 1907 he also headed a student organization, called the Wingolf, devoted to forming a Christian community, in which he found comfort from the isolation, he said, of having no university accommodation, college chaplain, or personal involvement with his teachers or their families. In 1909 he passed his first church board exam, completed his doctoral thesis on Schelling in 1910, began work as a vicar in Nauen in 1911, and in 1912 was ordained and qualified as a university lecturer. Soon after, through his sister, Johanna, and her husband, he met Grethi Wever whom he married in September 1914, just before volunteering for army service in the war.

Existentialism

The war completely changed Tillich. The change occurred suddenly one night, he said, in 1915. He linked it with what Kierkegaard, called an *Augenblick* – a "pregnant moment", said Tillich, "in which Eternity touches Time and demands a personal decision".[9] Tillich called it his "personal *kairos*". Something entirely new and unexpected on the instant broke into his life and radically transformed it. Together with his mother's death, the war made him acutely aware that life is finite. Writing to a friend, Maria Klein, the next year he said he had suddenly become aware that "It isn't only that *I* might die any day, but rather that everyone dies, *really* dies, you too".[10]

The war also overturned for him all traditional notions of God. It gave Him, Tillich said, "a demonic coloration".[11] It revealed "an abyss in human existence that could not be ignored".[12] Confronted with this abyss, Tillich was inspired by reading Nietzsche's ecstatic affirmation of existence. Faced with "the horror, ugliness and destructiveness of war",[13] Tillich was also inspired by art, particularly by a painting by Botticelli which he saw in Berlin towards the end of the war. It was a revelation, he wrote. So too was expressionist painting – the "breakthrough" of discovering "the creative ecstasy" of its destruction of form.[14] Through the war he had worked as an army chaplain on the Western

---

[9] Ibid. p. 61.

[10] Pauck p. 51.

[11] Tillich 1936 p. 33.

[12] Ibid. p. 52.

[13] Ibid. p. 27.

[14] Ibid. p. 28.

front, was awarded the Iron Cross First Class in June 1918, and ended his army service in Spandau. Then, when the war was over, he became a university teacher in Berlin and began developing his ideas about art and psychoanalysis, and about religious experience as the substance of culture which, he said, gives religious experience its form.

Meanwhile his wife, Grethi, whose child by him had died as a baby, became pregnant by one of his friends, Richard Wegener. She left Tillich and in June 1919 gave birth to Wegener's son, whom Tillich in a sense adopted by giving him his name. But he divorced Grethi. He now had several sexual liaisons, for which he was threatened with expulsion from the religious Wingolf society which he had joined and run as a student.

Then, on 5 January 1920, having early been bereaved of his mother, he suffered another loss, the death, in childbirth, of his sister, Johanna, with whom he had become very close after their mother's death. He became deeply depressed. To cheer him up, his other sister, Elisabeth, urged him to attend a Mardi Gras ball where he met an art teacher, Hannah Werner. She was ten years younger than him, and became very involved with him despite already being engaged to another man, Albert Gottschow, whom she married in Marburg that July. The next spring, however, she returned to Tillich, gave birth to Gottschow's son in June and after her divorce from Gottschow, married Tillich in March 1924.

Tillich now became interested, through Hannah, in poetry. He was particularly moved by what he called Rilke's "profound psychoanalytical realism, mystical richness, and a poetic form charged with metaphysical content".[15] He also became actively involved in politics. Mindful of social inequality since first starting school as a child, he wrote, the war made him also politically aware of the connection between capitalism and imperialism. Reading Marx, he said, also taught him how idealist philosophy serves the interests of those in power. How then was he to combine religious idealism with Marxism? Shortly after the 1917 Russian revolution he had sought to do so by joining a movement combining socialism and religion. With the German revolution of 1918 he turned increasingly to what he called a "sociologically based and politically oriented philosophy of history".[16] He wrote about socialism and Christianity and joined a group – later called the "*Kairos* circle" – which sought ways of restructuring society through attending to what is just and holy.

In a book published in 1923 he commended the pragmatist philosophy of William James and others. He also emphasized the human interest and

---

[15] Tillich 1936 p. 29.

[16] Ibid. p. 54.

need – including the need for meaning – which he maintained governs all science whether it is concerned with empirical reality, ideas, or the spirit. Like James, as I have said, he also emphasized personal experience. In doing so he was also influenced by the philosophy of Heidegger at Marburg University where he became professor of theology in 1924. He drew strongly on Heidegger's emphasis (published in his 1927 book, *Being and Time*) on the finite character of our existence, on the fact of our nothingness before and after life, and on the anxiety this causes us. Tillich called it "the relation of man to nothingness . . . fear of death, conscience, guilt, despair, daily life, loneliness".[17] They are all inherent in our being, our existence.

Not liking the restricted cultural life of Marburg, the Tillichs soon moved to Dresden where Paul became professor of philosophy and religious studies. The same year, 1925, saw the publication of his first popular book. In it he celebrated the revolt of nineteenth century philosophers against the materialist, self-sufficient individualism of capitalist culture and religion in favour of faith in God – in what Tillich called "the Unconditioned" – as the ultimate source of meaning and ground of being. In transcending the contingencies of empirical experience, he wrote, God can only be apprehended indirectly through what Tillich called "belief-ful realism". Belief in Him entails faith based on, and going beyond finite, real, material symbols mediating, representing, and conveying the spirit. Tillich rejected any collapse of one into the other – symbols into the spirit they represent. He also rejected the liberal notion of progress with its focus on the past and future to the neglect of the present which, in so far as it involves *kairos* is, said Tillich, "invaded by eternity".[18] It is this sense of the infinite, he claimed, apprehended through "unconscious, self-evident faith", which constitutes our "actual religious situation".[19]

Freud, he said, had been particularly important in the revolt of nineteenth century against capitalist materialism. For he had insisted on the distinction between body and spirit – between material and psychical reality – in developing psychoanalysis as a purely psychological form of therapy. Like religion, Tillich maintained, psychoanalysis sheds light both on "the demonic background of life" and on "the divine . . . the power which can sublimate the erotic drive present in all things psychical".[20]

---

[17] P. Tillich (1944) Existential philosophy, *Journal of the History of Ideas*, 5(1) January, pp. 44–70, 58.

[18] P. Tillich (1925) *The Religious Situation*, New York: Henry Holt, 1932, p. 176.

[19] Ibid. p. 40.

[20] Ibid. p. 62.

The next year, following the birth (on 17 February 1926) of their first child, Erdmuthe Christiane, the Tillichs holidayed in Paris. Here Paul completed a long essay,[21] in which he described the division of the conscious and unconscious mind as an example of what is demonic in contrast to the unity of what he defined as divine and holy. He also wrote of impulses within the unconscious as a source both of creativity and life, and of destruction in so far as they overwhelm consciousness, this only being resolvable, he said, through the infinite time of eternity and the divine.

In another essay he wrote more about time. He described "the timeless Logos" of Cartesian philosophy as "an immense abstraction". It does no justice, he said, to what he called the "decision of immediate existence", the *kairos*. He now described it as the moment when "time is disturbed by eternity" – a moment of ultimate meaning and revelation, free of the vagaries of chance.[22] At his inaugural lecture as professor of systematic theology in Leipzig, where he and his family moved in 1926, he spoke more about the idea of revelation, and in early 1928, at a conference in Crissier, near Geneva, he discussed its opposite – the divisions involved in the demonic.

The next year he was appointed to a professorship in theology in Frankfurt. Here, amongst other things, he supervised Adorno's doctoral dissertation on Kierkegaard's aesthetics, and helped Adorno and others found the Frankfurt Institute of Social Research. He was also very much involved with the arts and with politics. He helped start a socialist newspaper, and helped rescue left wing and Jewish students when, in July 1932, they were beaten up by Nazi storm troopers and students. He publicly demanded the expulsion of Nazi students from the university. As a result his next book, condemning the "barbarism" of the Nazis, was banned immediately after its publication. The following March, 1933, he was denounced in the *Frankfurter Zeitung* as the "embodiment of the enemy" because of his pro-Jewish and socialist sentiments and actions. The newspaper urged the university to purge itself of all such elements. On 13 April 1933 he was suspended but remained in Germany where, on 10 May, he witnessed the burning of books on the Nazi blacklist, including his own recently published book, *The Socialist Decision*.

Meanwhile Reinhold Niebuhr, professor of applied Christianity at New York's Union Theological Seminary, began negotiations for Tillich to be invited to a visiting professorship at Columbia. Wary of what he believed to be America's provincialism, Tillich nevertheless reluctantly accepted the resulting invitation.

----

[21] P. Tillich (1926) The demonic, in *The Interpretation of History*, New York: Scribner's, 1936, pp. 74–122.

[22] P. Tillich (1926) Kairos and Logos, ibid., pp. 123–75, 129.

He arrived in New York on 3 November 1933, and the next month learnt that he had been dismissed by the Nazis from his Frankfurt professorship. He now settled permanently in New York. His second child, René Stefan, was born (on 7 June 1935) and baptized there by Niebuhr. The next year, Tillich became chairman of a self-help organization founded that year for refugees like himself from central Europe. He also became involved with fellow refugees in a weekly discussion group at the New School for Social Research, where he also gave lectures.

Tillich's writing now included a brief autobiographical sketch in which he approved the work of both psychoanalysis and Marxism in seeking to unmask hidden levels of reality against defences driven by fear lest revelation of the truth destroy us.[23] He also wrote about his struggles with his father's authoritarian and dogmatic version of religion, and about culture becoming religious wherever it transcends human existence. Religious sacraments, he said, symbolize "the Unconditioned". But he also regretted their loss of meaning through failure to translate, as he put it, "the archaic language of liturgy and Scriptures into contemporary idiom".[24] His father was now ill with depression and old age and died in July 1937, leaving Tillich a ring inscribed, "Let the light shine in order that life may abound".[25] Earlier that year Tillich had been appointed to a permanent post as professor of philosophical theology at New York's Union Theological Seminary, and in March 1940 he became a US citizen.

At about the same time he became a member of Columbia University's Philosophy Club to which he gave a talk about existentialism which, through its January 1944 published version, became very influential. Tillich began it by allying German existentialism with US philosophy, specifically with the philosophy of William James. Just as William James prioritized experience over theory, he said, so too did the German proto-existentialists. They too distinguished between reality as an object of thinking and theorizing, and reality as immediately experienced. This philosophy, argued Tillich, originated in the writing of Schelling, Feuerbach, and Marx in the 1840s, and gained a new lease of life with the work of Nietzsche in the 1880s and with the pragmatist philosophy of William James at the beginning of the twentieth century.

Turning to religious experience, Tillich argued that existentialism and its nineteenth century precursors rejected Hegel's claim that essence and existence are the same in God and in man through the existence of the latter being

[23] Tillich 1936 p. 88.

[24] Ibid. p. 65.

[25] Pauck p. 264.

the "self-actualization of the Absolute".[26] We are not the same as God, insisted Tillich. Our existence is not the same. His is infinite, ours is limited. We cannot experience the infinity of His existence. We can only entertain it as an idea. To do so entails adopting the detachment described by Kierkegaard as characteristic of "the aesthetic attitude". Only through adopting this attitude can we relate to the possibility of a timeless essence in reality.[27]

Fromm emphasized that the task of the psychoanalyst, as of the Zen master, is to convey his being – "his existence". Tillich likewise emphasized that the existentialist does not seek to teach the truth as a separate object of knowledge. Rather, said Tillich,

> He can only create in his pupil by indirect communication that "Existential state" or personal experience out of which the pupil may think and act . . . the only possibility of educating is to bring the pupil by indirect methods to a personal experience of his own Existence.[28]

Furthermore, since existence – "*Dasein*", as Heidegger put it – can only be experienced, not known as something separate from us, it cannot be validly expressed as an object or thing. Heidegger accordingly sought alternative terms to express our being or existence. He emphasized the ontological, rather than the psychological character, of our anxiety about our nothingness before and after life. He also emphasized that, unlike other animals, we are the only mortal or "finite beings" who are aware of our mortality, of being finite.[29] Hence the importance of time in existentialism. Kierkegaard sought to escape its limited character in human existence, said Tillich, with his notion of the *Augenblick* – "the pregnant moment in which Eternity touches Time and demands a personal decision"[30] – which, as before, Tillich related to his Christian socialist notion of the *kairos*, the immediate personal experience of "the pregnant historical moment".[31]

But however transforming such a moment might be, we experience it alone. Our experience is personal to ourselves. Nevertheless, Tillich affirmed with Feuerbach that even our internal monologues consist of "a dialogue between the Ego and the Thou".[32] Furthermore, he said, as Marx pointed out, our loneliness

---

[26] P. Tillich (1944) Existential philosophy, *Journal of the History of Ideas* 5(1) pp. 44–70, 48.

[27] Ibid. p. 51.

[28] Ibid. p. 55.

[29] Ibid. p. 60.

[30] Ibid. p. 61.

[31] Ibid. p. 53.

[32] Ibid. p. 65.

is an effect of present historical conditions which can and should be changed. Existentialist philosophy has arisen because of the individualism and loneliness brought into being by capitalism in also reducing human beings to objects of "calculation and control",[33] thereby alienating people from themselves. At the same time religion declined as an effect of "enlightenment, social revolution, and bourgeois liberalism".[34] This resulted, said Tillich, in search for "an ultimate meaning of life", which existentialism discovered in immediate lived experience "prior to and beyond the distinction between objectivity and subjectivity".[35]

Just as Fromm later equated a return to non-distinction between subject and object with Buddhist enlightenment, Tillich equated it with mystical experience. But, he insisted, for the existentialist this does not mean "mystical union with the transcendent Absolute". Rather it means "faith toward union with the depth of life".[36] Putting this historically, Tillich argued that existentialism seeks:

> Return to a pre-Cartesian attitude, to an attitude in which the sharp gulf between the subjective and the objective "realms" had not yet been created, and the essence of objectivity could be found in the depth of subjectivity – in which God could be best approached through the soul.[37]

In thus situating existentialism historically, Tillich argued that the reason it had not arisen in England, as it had in other European countries between 1830 and 1930, was because England did not suffer a decline in religion at that time. Perhaps he meant that God was so much part of the furniture of England's established church that there was little impetus to pronounce Him either alive or dead. Whatever the reason, the British philosopher, G. E. Moore, was bemused by Tillich's talk. When it came to his turn to comment on it, he said, "Now really, Mr. Tillich, I don't think I have been able to understand a single sentence of your paper".[38]

Much more comprehensible – indeed it won Tillich a very large following – was his relating existentialism to religion in his post-war Union Theological Seminary sermons. Particularly notable was a sermon he finished writing on his sixtieth birthday, on 20 August 1946.

....

33 Ibid. p. 66.

34 Ibid. p. 66.

35 Ibid. p. 67.

36 Ibid. p. 67.

37 Ibid. p. 67.

38 In Pauck p. 313 n. 96.

Transforming acceptance

Tillich began the sermon, "You are accepted", by dwelling on sin. He equated it with separation from oneself, from others, and from what he called "the Ground of Being".[39] Unlike other animals, he argued, we not only suffer from separation. In separation, he said, "We know that we are estranged from something to which we really belong, and with which we *should* be united".[40] We first learn of separation in being separated from our mothers on being born. Experiencing it – like William James' father experiencing Swedenborgian "vastation" – is the precondition of the healing of the divided self into oneness. Tillich put it in terms of the sin of separation being healed through grace, through "the *re*union of life with life".[41]

He also described self-separation psychoanalytically, in terms of separation between what is conscious and unconscious. He also quoted St Paul describing as sin the self-estrangement in which one feels "if I should do what I do not wish to do, it is not I that do it, but rather sin which dwells within me".[42] He then described St Paul's transforming experience of God on the road to Damascus:

> In the picture of Jesus as the Christ, which appeared to him at the moment of his greatest separation from other men, from himself and God, he found himself accepted in spite of his being rejected. And when he found that he was accepted, he was able to accept himself and to be reconciled to others.[43]

A similar experience of being accepted by someone else – human or divine – lies at the heart, suggested Tillich, of all transformation from what he called the sin of separation to the grace of reunion. One cannot will it. Emphasizing the point, he wrote:

> We cannot transform our lives, unless we allow them to be transformed by that stroke of grace. It happens; or it does not happen. . . . It strikes us when we feel that our separation is deeper than usual, because we have violated another life, a life which we loved, or from which we were estranged. It strikes us when our disgust for our own being, our indifference, our weakness, our hostility, and our lack of direction and composure have become intolerable to us. . . . Sometimes at that moment a wave of light breaks into our darkness, and it is as though a voice were saying: "You are accepted. *You are accepted*, accepted by that which is greater than you, and the name of which you do not know. Do not ask for the name now . . . Do not seek for anything; do not perform anything; do not intend

---

39 P. Tillich (1946) You are accepted, in Tillich 1949, pp. 155–65, 156.

40 Ibid. p. 157.

41 Ibid. p. 158.

42 Ibid. pp. 160–1.

43 Ibid. p. 162.

anything. *Simply accept the fact that you are accepted!* If that happens to us, we experience grace. . . . And nothing is demanded of this experience, no religious or moral or intellectual presupposition, nothing but *acceptance*.[44]

With this the "sin" of threefold separation – from oneself, from others, from God or the Ground of Being – is healed. Through transforming grace we are reunited with ourselves and "accept the life of another" knowing that their life "belongs to the same Ground to which we belong, and by which we have been accepted".[45] Feeling accepted by what is greater than us makes us love life in ourselves and others because of the certainty such acceptance gives us of "the eternal meaning of our life".[46] Saying "yes" to life can bring us peace in making us whole. "Then", concluded Tillich, "we can say that grace has come upon us".[47]

Tillich wrote more along these lines in a book which he had begun many years before in Marburg. Writing about therapy in the book's first volume, he linked it to his newly developing theory about being accepted. Putting this in religious terms, he wrote:

> He who knows God or the Christ in the sense of being grasped by him and being united with him does the good. He who knows the essential structure of things in the sense of having received their meaning and power acts according to them; he does the good, even if he has to die for it.[48]

Psychoanalysis teaches the same. It teaches the healing power of insight, of transforming oneness with one's past. But Tillich also distinguished between psychoanalysis and religion. Religion, he said, deals with anxiety about our nothingness due to the finite character of our existence. Psychoanalysis deals with compulsive fear of objects onto which we displace this anxiety about death and nothingness.

Final courage

Tillich popularized these ideas in a book, *The Courage to Be*. In it he insisted that the courage of being entails also facing its opposite – the finality of our non-being, mortality, and death – of which the supreme example, he said, was Socrates.[49] Embracing non-being entails stripping both death and life of the

---

44 Ibid. pp. 163–4.

45 Ibid. p. 164.

46 Ibid. p. 164.

47 Ibid. p. 165.

48 P. Tillich (1951) *Systematic Theology, Vol. I*, Welwyn: James Nisbet, 1953, p. 107.

49 For a moving account of Socrates' death see Plato (n.d.), *Phaedo*, in *The Last Days of Socrates*, Harmondsworth: Penguin, 1954, pp. 97–183.

masks with which we defend against nothingness. It is these masks that cause us neurotic, as opposed to existential, anxiety.

> Our [neurotic] anxiety puts frightening masks over all men and things. If we strip them of these masks their own countenance appears and the fear they produce disappears. This is true even of death . . . . The horrors connected with it are a matter of imagination. They vanish when the mask is taken from the image of death. It is our uncontrolled desires that create masks and put them over men and things.[50]

We defend against life and death, the nothingness of non-being, with fantasies and dreams, feared by Hamlet in his soliloquy, "To be or not to be". Nor is it any wonder we thus defend against the anxiety of the nothingness or non-being that is a corollary of our being if, as Tillich claimed

> It is impossible for a finite being to stand naked anxiety for more than a flash of time. People who have experienced these moments, as for instance some mystics in their visions of the "night of the soul", or Luther under the despair of the demonic assaults, or Nietzsche-Zarathustra in the experience of the "great disgust", have told of the unimaginable horror of it.[51]

To avoid the horror we try to transform fear of nothingness into fear of something. Phobia is a case in point. So too is the panic fear described by William James in *The Varieties of Religious Experience*. But transforming fear of nothing into fear of something cannot do away with our nothingness. For our nothingness is inherent in the finite character of our human existence. It cannot be escaped. In neurosis we try to escape it by putting an imaginary world in its place. But this leads to misplaced feelings of safety, certainty, fear, and guilt.

We can only truly overcome guilt, Tillich maintained, through affirming and taking on ourselves the anxiety belonging to the destructiveness of our split-off demonic depth. And this entails recognizing our participation in something beyond ourselves. In psychoanalysis, said Tillich, overcoming guilt is achieved through the patient participating in the healing power of the therapist accepting him despite the patient's feeling that he is unacceptable. In this the therapist does not stand for himself but for acceptance which has to be embodied in a particular person who alone, wrote Tillich, "can realize guilt, who can judge, and who can accept in spite of the judgement".[52]

Ultimately, Tillich claimed, acceptance rests with God. It depends on "being-itself". It depends on accepting God's acceptance. And this entails faith in

---

[50] P. Tillich (1952) *The Courage to Be*, Glasgow: Collins, pp. 24–5.

[51] Ibid. p. 47.

[52] Ibid. p. 161.

being grasped by His being bridging the gap between what is finite and infinite. It depends on accepting, as Tillich put it, that "he who is separated is accepted".[53] On this rests our courage to be and our courage to take on the anxieties of fate, death, guilt, blame, emptiness, and meaninglessness, exacerbated by the rational calculation and control of science and technology seemingly doing away with the meaningfulness of our existence.

Many were so taken with Tillich's account of being accepted that they looked to him for therapy. He also now became very much in demand as a speaker. Like William James he too gave a series of Gifford Lectures – in Aberdeen in 1953 and 1954. He became so popular as a lecturer that a talk he gave in January 1960 in Berkeley – on the immortality of the soul – attracted a crowd of over three thousand. Intrigued, like Fromm, by Buddhist mysticism, he went to Japan for a couple of months that summer. On his return to America he wrote of the importance of submitting all religions to what he called "the criterion of faith which transcends every finite symbol of faith and the ultimate criterion of a love which unconditionally affirms, judges, and receives the other person".[54]

Writing further about love, therapy, and religion, he compared the impact of religious sacraments via the unconscious on consciousness with the influence of the unconscious in encounters between patients and therapists, and between lovers and their beloved. Protestantism, he said, fearful of religious sacraments becoming demonic through bypassing consciousness and the consent of the will, had wrongly minimized the rites of religion, thereby rendering spirit merely a matter of morality and reason. Psychoanalysis, by contrast, restored credence to the spirit through its recognition of the unconscious. If the church did not also take account of the need to free the spirit from mind and matter it risked becoming obsolete. It also needed to stop its nay-saying – in the name of saintliness – to drinking, dancing, and so on. Again psychoanalysis was relevant, he said, for it affirms both sex and love. It thereby challenges the moralizing of both Christianity and humanism. It demonstrates, said Tillich, that "even the most sublime functions of the spirit are rooted in the vital trends of human nature".[55]

Tillich wrote this in the third volume of his book, *Systematic Theology*. It does not make easy reading. His popular books, however, made him a household name. Together with other intellectuals he attended White House

---

[53] Ibid. p. 161.

[54] P. Tillich (1960) On the boundary line, *Christian Century*, 77(4) pp. 1435–7, 1435.

[55] P. Tillich (1963) *Systematic Theology, Vol. III*, Welwyn: James Nisbet, 1964, p. 255.

celebrations of the inauguration of President Kennedy. In 1963 he was invited to contribute to the fortieth anniversary celebrations of *Time* magazine (in which he had been lauded, with his picture on the front cover, in March 1959). In his contribution to the magazine's anniversary celebration, Tillich encouraged his audience to transcend the drive towards endlessly increasing material production through uniting with what he called "creation".[56] When he died a couple of years later, on 22 October 1965, his death was announced on radio, TV, and in a long obituary on the front page of the *New York Times*. Subsequently, as I indicated at the outset of this chapter, there have been reasons to take issue with his theology. Nevertheless, the existentialism of his approach to religion and psychoanalysis has proved enormously fruitful, particularly as developed by Viktor Frankl, as I will now discuss.

---

[56] P. Tillich (1963) The ambiguity of perfection, *Time*, 17 May, p. 69.

Chapter 7

Viktor Frankl

Logotherapy

Viktor Frankl's existentialist "logotherapy" version of therapy has proved immensely popular. It is also regarded, by many, as an arch synthesis of religion and psychoanalysis. Frankl did indeed combine notions about God and the unconscious. He wrote less about God, however, than about the spirit, and in no way did he adopt the attention of Freud and other psychoanalysts to fantasy accessed through free association and the transference and counter-transference relation of analyst and patient in analysis. Indeed his somewhat quick-fix method of therapy – particularly his advocacy of "paradoxical intention" and behaviour modification, which I will return to later in this chapter – involves not so much analysis as treatment through suggestion. Furthermore, he entirely rejected Freud's emphasis on infantile sexuality and biological instinct.

His preferred emphasis on spirituality has contributed to making his work much more popular than many other versions of religion and psychoanalysis. By the early 1990s the *New York Times* reported that his book, *Man's Search for Meaning*, was one of the ten most influential books in America. It is also influential well beyond America. Despite the somewhat unappealing, self-congratulatory tone of Frankl's writing, his work is deservedly influential. In my view at least, he rightly emphasized that health involves recognizing our responsibility, freedom of choice, and meaning in our existence oriented by love of what is good outside and beyond us. I will detail all this, perhaps somewhat over-repetitively, in seeking to become clear about it myself after first recounting Frankl's early life and work in Vienna.

Viennese youth

Frankl's spiritually centred approach to therapy has been dubbed the third Viennese school of psychotherapy. Like Freud and Adler, the founders in Vienna of psychoanalysis and psychoanalytically-based individual psychology, Viktor Frankl was brought up in Vienna. He was born there – in Czerningasse – across the street from where Adler once lived. Like Freud and Adler, Frankl too was Jewish. His family kept a kosher kitchen, fasted on Yom Kippur, and prayed daily. But they were not strictly orthodox.[1] Viktor went to the same secondary school as Freud had attended over thirty years before. Whilst there he became interested in psychoanalysis and by his teens, he later bragged, he had already formulated the two central tenets of his logotherapy approach to therapy: first, that we should not ask the meaning of life but rather what life asks of us; and second, that the ultimate meaning of our existence lies beyond our understanding but must be believed in, even if only unconsciously.[2]

Whilst still a teenager, he also bragged, he sent an essay (about bodily movements signifying sexual assent and disgust) to Freud who arranged for its publication.[3] In 1925 Frankl also became involved with Adler's school of psychoanalysis, but soon abandoned it because of Adler's psychological reductionism. He also helped organize youth counselling centres in various cities including Vienna where, in 1928, he got a job working in a centre for people suffering with depression. It was here, Frankl later said, that he first developed his logotherapy tenet that we find meaning in life through changing our attitude to fate; through choosing, making, and doing; and through love.

After qualifying as a doctor, in 1930, he worked in Vienna University's psychiatric clinic and in 1932 he became director of a unit for suicidal patients in a psychiatric hospital – the Steinhof. Here, he later wrote, he learnt to distinguish between those who were and those who were not seriously intent on killing themselves in terms of whether they said they could not die because they had a duty or meaning to fulfil. If they had a duty or meaning to fulfil it was safe to discharge them because, he said, quoting Nietzsche, "He who has a 'Why' to live can endure any 'How'".[4]

Following the German invasion of Vienna in March 1938 Frankl became chief neurologist in Vienna's then only Jewish hospital. Here he was again involved in saving people from suicide, but in a situation which was now so bleak for Jews that increasing numbers sought to kill themselves. To save them from the Nazi edict ordering the destruction, through euthanasia, of all mentally ill patients, Frankl diagnosed patients admitted to his unit as physically, not mentally, ill. The same year, 1938, he coined the term "existential

[1] H. Klingberg (2001) *When Life Calls Out to Us: The Love and Lifework of Viktor and Elly Frankl*, New York: Doubleday, pp. 28–9.

[2] V. Frankl (1995) *Recollections*, Cambridge, Mass: Perseus, 2000, p. 56.

[3] V. Frankl (1924) Zur mimischen Bejahung und Verneinung, *Internationale Zeitschrift für Psychoanalyse*, **10** pp. 437–8, abstracted by J. Flugel (1925) General, *IJPA*, **6** p. 462.

[4] In Klingberg p. 122.

analysis" to describe his method of therapy.[5] Soon after, in the early months of the war, he met a nurse, Tilly Grosser, whom he married in 1941. Although he obtained a US visa, they remained in Vienna where Viktor began work on a book, *Ärztliche Seelsorge* (later translated as *The Doctor and the Soul*) which apparently comforted one of his friends, Hubert Suer, when he was imprisoned and condemned to death by the Nazis. Soon Frankl too was imprisoned.

Concentration camp experiences

In 1942 Viktor Frankl, who had remained in Vienna to be with his family, was deported with them to Thereisenstadt near Prague. Here Viktor's 81-year-old father, Gabriel, died from starvation, pulmonary edema, and pneumonia. Soon after Viktor's mother, Elsa, was sent to Auschwitz where she was immediately sent to the gas chambers. Viktor's older brother, Walter, also died in Auschwitz, in a mine in one of its camps. Only their younger sister, Stella, who went to Australia, survived.

Like their mother, Viktor too was sent to Auschwitz. His wife, Tilly, was granted two years' dispensation from deportation because of her work in a munitions factory, but she chose to go too to be with Viktor. They were separated at the camp. Initially, Viktor later recalled, he only survived through luck. On his arrival the notorious Dr Joseph Mengele directed him to go to the right, but since Viktor did not know anyone there he went to the left, where he saw some of his junior colleagues. Had he not done so, he said, he would certainly have been sent to the gas chambers. "Only God knows," he later wrote, "where I got that idea or found the courage".[6]

In the lining of his coat he had the draft of his book, *The Doctor and the Soul*. But it was lost when he and his fellow-inmates had to throw everything they had on the ground. In place of his coat Viktor found another one – old and torn – with a piece of paper in the pocket on which was written the Jewish prayer, the *Shema Israel*, "Hear, oh Israel, the Lord our God is One". He kept it as a talisman, hidden in his coat as he had previously concealed the draft of his book.

The idea of the book saved him, he said. Wanting to finish it gave him a purpose, a sense of meaning. From Auschwitz he was sent to Kaufering III and then to Türkheim near Munich. Here, he later said:

> I am convinced that I owe my survival, among other things, to my resolve to reconstruct that lost manuscript. I started to work on it when I was sick with typhus and

[5] V. Frankl (1938) Zur Geistigen Problematik der Psychotherapie, *Zeitschrift für Psychotherapie*, **10** pp. 33–45.

[6] Frankl 1995 p. 93.

tried to keep awake, even in the night, to prevent a vascular collapse. For my fortieth birthday [on 26 March 1945] an inmate had given me a pencil stub, and almost miraculously he had pilfered a few small SS forms. On the backs of these forms I scribbled notes that might help me reconstruct *The Doctor and the Soul*.[7]

Others kept other talismans. An example was a Dutch labourer Frankl met when he was walking away, across a field, on his release from Türkheim. The man kept playing with a small object which Frankl asked him to show him. Thereupon the man opened his hand to reveal "a tiny golden globe, the oceans painted in blue enamel, with a gold band for the equator . . . [with the] inscription: 'The whole world turns on love'".[8] It was just like a pendant Viktor had given Tilly on her first birthday with him. Perhaps, Frankl speculated, it was the only other pendant like it in the world. Certainly there had only ever been two such pendants in Vienna.

But Tilly was dead. The first morning after his return to Vienna, Viktor learnt that she had died at Bergen-Belsen. Following its liberation 17,000 corpses were found there. To these were added, over the next six weeks, another 17,000 deaths of prisoners from sickness, starvation, and exhaustion, of whom Tilly, it seems, was one. Meanwhile, in Vienna, Viktor was appointed to head the Polyclinic's neurology department (where he worked for the next twenty-five years). He was also urged to complete the book he had begun before the war so as to qualify as a university lecturer. Finishing the book was a godsend. It gave him something to do. So too did dictating – in just nine days, he said – another book, *Ein Psycholog erlebt das Konzentrationslager*, describing his concentration camp experiences.

Both books were published in 1946. The same year Viktor met a 20-year-old Catholic nurse, Eleonore Katharina Schwindt, whom he married the next July 1947 (after confirmation the same week of Tilly's death). Their only child, Gabriele, was born that December. The next year Viktor's third book, *Der unbewusste Gott*, was published. This was followed, in 1955, by the publication of another book, *Pathologie des Zeitgestes*, in which Frankl described people suffering what he called an "existential vacuum". Soon after the Harvard psychologist, Gordon Allport – author of a book, published in 1956, called *The Individual and his Religion* – helped persuade a publisher to publish Frankl's 1946 book about his concentration camp experiences in English.

It resulted in Frankl's most famous book, *Man's Search for Meaning*. It begins with Frankl's account of the shock he and his fellow-inmates experienced on

---

[7] Frankl 1995 p. 98.

[8] Ibid. p. 91.

first arriving in the concentration camp. He then described in much more detail their subsequent experience of meaninglessness. He described this – and the apathy involved – as "a kind of emotional death".[9] Life in the camps, he said, became reduced to preoccupation with food and physical comfort. Prisoners dreamt of nothing but "bread, cake, cigarettes, and nice warm baths".[10] They lost all interest in sex. Some however retained their religious belief. It was, said Frankl, "the most sincere imaginable".[11] They retreated from their terrible surroundings to a life of inner richness and spiritual freedom.

Frankl's own spiritual recovery came through love. He described it transforming him suddenly early one morning on being force-marched to work:

> We stumbled on in the darkness, over big stones and through large puddles, along the one road leading from the camp. The accompanying guards kept shouting at us and driving us with the butts of their rifles. Anyone with very sore feet supported himself on his neighbor's arm. Hardly a word was spoken; the icy wind did not encourage talk. Hiding his mouth behind his upturned collar, the man marching next to me whispered suddenly: "If our wives could see us now! I do hope they are better off in their camps and don't know what is happening to us. That brought thoughts of my own wife to mind. . . . my mind clung to my wife's image, imagining it with an uncanny acuteness. I heard her answering me, saw her smile, her frank and encouraging look. Real or not, her look was then more luminous than the sun which was beginning to rise. A thought transfixed me: for the first time in my life I saw the truth as it is set into song by so many poets, proclaimed as the final wisdom by so many thinkers. The truth – that love is the ultimate and the highest goal to which man can aspire. Then I grasped the meaning of the greatest secret that human poetry and human thought and belief have to impart: *The salvation of man is through love and in love.* I understood how a man who has nothing left in this world still may know bliss, be it only for a brief moment, in the contemplation of his beloved. In a position of utter desolation, when man cannot express himself in positive action, when his only achievement may consist in enduring his sufferings in the right way – an honorable way – in such a position man can, through living contemplation of the image he carries of his beloved, achieve fulfillment. . . . A thought crossed my mind: I didn't even know if she were still alive. I knew only one thing – which I have learned well by now: Love goes very far beyond the physical person of the beloved. It finds its deepest meaning in his spiritual being, his inner self. Whether or not he is actually present, whether or not he is still alive at all, ceases somehow to be of importance.[12]

Intensified spiritual belief in something or someone loved and good beyond them helped prisoners survive their otherwise spiritually empty lives. As their belief in their inner life and spirit returned they experienced the beauty of art

---

[9] V. Frankl (1959) *Man's Search for Meaning*, London: Hodder & Stoughton, 1964, p. 18.

[10] Ibid. p. 27.

[11] Ibid. p. 33.

[12] Ibid. pp. 35–7.

and nature as never before. Without this many were reduced to animal mean-inglessness. They became frightened of making any decisions. They succumbed to feeling fate was their master. Against this outcome Frankl insisted that, even despite the oppression of camp life, it was still possible to maintain "a vestige of spiritual freedom", to "choose one's attitude . . . one's own way".[13] He quoted Dostoevsky: "There is one thing that I dread: not to be worthy of my sufferings".[14]

An example of someone in the camps who achieved just such worth, he said, was a young woman. She was dying and thanked fate for hitting her so hard. Before, she said, when life had been easy for her, she had not taken spiritual achievement seriously. Now she did. Pointing through the window of the hut where she lay, she said, "This tree here is the only friend I have in my loneliness . . . I often talk to this tree". And did the tree reply, asked Frankl. "Yes . . . It said to me, 'I am here – I am here – I am life, eternal life'".[15]

Others lost their spirit. They became victims, said Frankl, of the camp's "degenerating influences".[16] Everything became meaningless. For them therapy entailed giving them back their spirit. It entailed enabling them to recover a future to choose to look forward to. In this context Frankl quoted Spinoza: "Emotion, which is suffering, ceases to be suffering as soon as we form a clear and precise picture of it".[17] For one suicidal prisoner recovery occurred through his being reminded of the child he adored who was waiting for him in another country. For another suicidal inmate – a scientist – recovery entailed having pointed out to him that he had written a series of books which still needed finishing.

One evening, when all the prisoners were feeling particularly depressed because they had been starved all day as punishment for not saying who it was who had stolen potatoes from the store, Frankl was asked, as a psychiatrist, to say something that might help. He reminded them that they still had a great deal to look forward to. He quoted Nietzsche: "That which does not kill me, makes me stronger".[18] He reminded them of their hopes for the future, and of their joys from the past. He quoted the writings of a poet, "What you have experienced, no power on earth can take from you".[19] Somebody looks down

---

[13] V. Frankl (1959) *Man's Search for Meaning*, London: Hodder & Stoughton, 1964, p. 65.

[14] Ibid. p. 66.

[15] Ibid. p. 69.

[16] Ibid. p. 69.

[17] Ibid. p. 74.

[18] Ibid. p. 82.

[19] Ibid. pp. 82–3.

on us in difficult times, he said, "a friend, a wife, somebody alive or dead, or a God".[20] They would not expect us to disappoint them. They would want to find us suffering proudly – not miserably. They would want us to know how to die. He told them about a friend who, when he arrived at the camp, sought to make a pact with heaven that his suffering and death would save the person he loved from a painful end. For him suffering and death were meaningful. He did not want to die for nothing. Nobody does.

Detailing this in his book, Frankl went on to describe his fellow-prisoners' experience after their liberation. At the end of the first day one asked another, "Tell me, were you pleased today?" Shame-facedly the other replied, "No". They had "lost the ability to feel pleased," said Frankl. "Everything appeared unreal, unlikely, as in a dream. We could not believe it was true".[21] A few days later, walking in the country, hearing the joy of larks rising with nothing but the wide earth and sky around, Frankl fell to his knees with the thought, always the same, "I called to the Lord from my narrow prison and He answered me in the freedom of space".[22] It was then, he said, that his new life started. It was then that he became a human being again.

But bitterness could recur: bitterness when the newly freed prisoner felt others did not fully acknowledge what he had been through, when he wondered what it had all been for. Or he could feel bitterly disillusioned on discovering that, after all the suffering he had been through, there was more suffering to come: the suffering, for instance, of having lost or losing those he loved. Frankl ended his book, however, with reviving religious experience: "The crowning experience of all, for the homecoming man," he said, "is the wonderful feeling that, after all he has suffered, there is nothing he need fear any more – except his God".[23]

Spiritual meaning

In a 1962 supplement to his book about his concentration camp experiences Frankl explained his theory of logotherapy, of therapy through spiritual meaning. Whereas, he said, Freud and Adler emphasized the will to pleasure and power, he emphasized "the will to meaning". The meaning of our lives is not something we invent, he said. It is something we discover. It may involve a cause to which we commit ourselves for the sake of God or for the sake of someone we love.

---

[20] Ibid. p. 83.

[21] Ibid. p. 88.

[22] Ibid. p. 90.

[23] Ibid. p. 93.

He went on to discuss ways this commitment can be thwarted. He talked of "existential frustration", using the term "existential" to denote what is specifically human (as opposed to animal) in our being and existing. It involves taking responsibility for finding a concrete meaning in our lives. Frustration of this goal is not necessarily pathological. But it can lead to spiritual malaise. Frankl called it "noölogical neurosis". It is not well served by Freudian therapy focusing on returning patients to meaningless, instinctual, animal forces in their unconscious. Rather noölogical neurosis calls for focus on what is meaningful. It calls for attention to the reality of the spirit. Contrasting his approach to therapy with that of Freud, Frankl wrote:

> Logotherapy deviates from psychoanalysis insofar as it considers man as a being whose main concern consists in fulfilling a meaning and in actualizing values, rather than in the mere gratification and satisfaction of drives and instincts, or in merely reconciling the conflicting claims of id, ego and superego, or in the mere adaptation and adjustment to society and environment.[24]

It is because our will to meaning is thwarted that we may become preoccupied with pleasure or power. This preoccupation is a by-product of existential frustration. It is an effect rather than a cause of spiritual – noölogical – neurosis.

Ultimately, Frankl emphasized, as he had before, it is not so much the meaning of our life that we should discover but rather what life asks of us. Logotherapy, he added, seeks to make its patients aware of their responsibility. It accordingly leaves it to the patient to discover for what or to whom he is responsible. Many feel themselves to be responsible and accountable to God. They interpret their lives both in terms of a task to be done, and in terms of a divine taskmaster beyond them who has set it.

The logotherapist, said Frankl, should enable patients to become aware of meaning in the world beyond them. Whereas some therapists advocate self-actualization, Frankl advocated self-transcendence through outwardly-directed doing, being, and loving. Love is the only way of experiencing someone else in the spiritual core of their being. Influenced by Heidegger, Frankl argued that love enables us to see what is not yet actualized, but ought to be actualized, in the person we love. Through love we enable the beloved to actualize what is as yet only potential within them.

Love may reveal to us meaning in suffering. To illustrate all this Frankl cited the case of an elderly doctor who consulted him on account of severe depression following the death of his wife. What would have happened if his wife had survived him, Frankl asked. "Oh," said the doctor, "for her this would have

---

[24] V. Frankl (1962) Basic concepts of logotherapy, in Frankl, 1959 pp. 97–137, 105.

been terrible; how she would have suffered!" At this Frankl pointed out, "You see, Doctor, such a suffering has been spared her, and it was you who have spared her this suffering; but now, you have to pay for it by surviving and mourning her".[25] Suffering, he concluded, ceases to be suffering as soon as it finds a meaning.

Another example was a woman in group therapy who, following the death of her 11-year-old son, tried to kill herself because she could not face coping on her own with looking after his older brother who had been paralyzed since infancy. Turning to a young woman in the group, Frankl asked her to imagine herself when she was 80 dying after a successful and wealthy but childless life. At this the young woman saw herself looking back regretting her lack of children. Frankl then invited the first patient – the would-be suicide – similarly to imagine looking back on her life. At this she burst into tears. She saw that her life would not be a failure. It would be full of meaning from having done her best for her paralyzed son.

Turning next to the feeling that life is meaningless because it is so transient and finite, Frankl argued that all that is transient is our possibilities. As soon as we realize them they are rescued from transience by becoming concrete. The transience of our existence does not render it meaningless. But it does entail our responsibility for realizing what is otherwise only possible and potential. Early on in his 1962 supplement to *Man's Search for Meaning* he had remarked that, whereas in previous times people sought spiritual help from pastors, priests, or rabbis, they now sought spiritual help from doctors or psychiatrists. He ended this supplement by warning against what he had previously called an existential vacuum. He described the loss of meaningfulness involved as the collective neurosis of our time. He also warned against reductively explaining people in terms of their biology, psychology, or social conditions. For this, he said, overlooks the fact that our existence is not mechanically determined but freely chosen. Existing involves choosing from one moment to the next what will become of us. Nor is religious experience psychodynamically determined as Freud maintained. It too is a matter of choice.

An example was a 60-year-old man who, for many decades, had suffered auditory hallucinations:

> Everyone in his environment regarded him as an idiot. Yet what a strange charm radiated from this man! As a child he had wanted to become a priest. However, he had to be content with the only joy he could experience, and that was singing in the church choir on Sunday mornings. Now, his sister who accompanied him reported that

---

[25] Ibid. p. 115.

> sometimes he grew very excited; yet in the last moment he was always able to regain his self-control.[26]

Why did he do this? – because of fixation to his sister? No. When Frankl asked him for whom he did it he replied, "For God's sake". His answer demonstrated, said Frankl, his authentic, self-chosen religious life deep within him.

Doctor and soul

By now Frankl's work was so successful that, in 1965, the book, *Ärztliche Seelsorge* (*The Doctor and the Soul*), which he had written before, during, and after his concentration camp experiences, was issued in English. Frankl dedicated it to the memory of his first wife, Tilly. It begins with his observation that people no longer look so much to priests as to doctors for spiritual help. Doctors, or at least therapists, he said, might therefore do well to rest their faith in religion as an anchor in their life. He went on to emphasize the spirituality, free choice, and responsibility distinguishing us from animals driven by instinct, heredity, and environment. Therapy should seek to enable people to become free of being similarly driven. It should attend to its patients' spirituality, not adjust their biologically-given drives to external reality, as advocated by Freud, nor oppose the will of the ego to the demands of the id, as advocated by Adler.

Since the end of the nineteenth century, Frankl argued, people have been portrayed as driven by psychological and social forces. By contrast existentialism recognizes and asserts our freedom in face of these forces. It restores consciousness and responsibility to the heart of our existence. He quoted the existentialist philosopher and psychiatrist, Karl Jaspers, describing man not as someone who just "is", but as someone who is a "deciding" being. He decides "what is".[27]

Whereas psychoanalysis seeks to bring instinct to consciousness, logotherapy seeks to bring spiritual reality – particularly responsibility – to consciousness. Its starting point is consciousness of responsibility. But what we are responsible for can only be discovered in terms of the specific meaning of each person's life. Our life's transience does not make it meaningless. Through actualizing our possibilities we safely establish them for all eternity. Logotherapy accordingly seeks to enable patients to become conscious of, and responsible for realizing their unique and singular possibilities. Some, Frankl said, go further. They feel the life tasks they are responsible for fulfilling come from God.

---

[26] V. Frankl (1962) Basic concepts of logotherapy, in Frankl, 1959 p. 135.

[27] V. Frankl (1965) *The Doctor and the Soul*, New York: Vintage Books, 1973 p. 21.

Since we are finite, since we are mortal, we cannot endlessly postpone choosing and doing. Our mortality entails our responsibility for deciding what to make of each and every moment of our life. At no moment can we escape the responsibility of choosing between possibilities. Our being in the world – and here Frankl used Heidegger's term *Dasein* – entails that we are always free to choose the nature of our being. Our responsibility consists in realizing our being through doing, experiencing, and suffering. A prime example, given by Heidegger and repeated by Frankl, is the examining magistrate in Tolstoy's novella, *The Death of Ivan Ilyich*, whose existence is redeemed and illuminated at the end by his choosing to accept the pain of his dying, and by choosing not to cause his family any more suffering.

Meaning is not acquired through absence of suffering. It does not come from pleasure, nor from taking drugs. They simply numb us to awareness and consciousness of our unhappiness. Suppressing feeling because it is unpleasant kills our inner life. Suffering and trouble belong to life. So too do fate and death. They cannot be taken away from life without destroying its meaning. Nor can the past. Rather accepting, grieving, and repenting for it enables us to take hold of the past so as to recognize ourselves as its authors, not simply its meaningless victims. Whilst psychoanalysis aims to enable patients to become capable of pleasure, existential therapy may have to settle for enabling people to become capable of suffering. Indeed suffering, illness, and death can, paradoxically, bring people alive to their ultimate existential capacities. To highlight the point Frankl again cited the example of the young woman dying in the concentration camp saying of a chestnut tree outside her window, of which she could only see a single twig with a couple of blossoms, that it said to her "I am here, I am here – I am life, eternal life".[28] She met her fate, Frankl indicated, by choosing to accept it.

Acceptance is an act of will. Exercising our will, we are no longer degraded to a mere means of economic and biological production and reproduction. Our dignity forbids it. The opposite of such degradation is love. It recognizes the spiritual being of the other:

> In love the beloved person is comprehended in his very essence, as the unique and singular being that he is; he is comprehended as a Thou, and as such is taken into the self . . . . The person who is loved "can't help" having the uniqueness and singularity of his self – that is, the value of his personality – realized. Love is not deserved, is unmerited – it is simply grace.[29]

---

28 Ibid. p. 115.

29 Ibid. pp. 132–3.

Whereas sexual attraction and infatuation address what the other person "has" – their physical and psychological characteristics – love addresses what the other person "is".

Perhaps thinking of his mindfulness, in the concentration camp, of his love of his first wife, Tilly, not knowing whether she was alive or dead, Frankl went on:

> Love is an intentional act. What it intends is the essence of the other person. This essence is ultimately independent of existence . . . That is why love can outlast the death of the beloved. The existence of the beloved can be annihilated by death, but his essence cannot be touched by death.[30]

Frankl illustrated the point with the example of a fellow concentration camp prisoner who said that whenever time and conditions in the camp allowed he thought about his mother. He held imaginary dialogues with her. At such times, he said, "the fact that I did not even know whether she was alive hardly disturbed me".[31]

Truly comprehending the inner nature of another person by seeing them in the illumination of love is akin to recognizing truth as eternal. Or, as another writer quoted by Frankl puts it, "love sees a person the way God 'meant' him".[32] Psychotherapists, said Frankl, should similarly seek to see their patients in terms of their most personal possibilities. Expanding the point, he added:

> Love permits us to see the spiritual core of the other person, the reality of the other's essential nature and his value potentialities. Love allows us to experience another's personality as a world in itself, and so extends our own world. While it thus enriches and "requites" us, it also does the other person good in leading him to those potential values which can be seen and anticipated only in love. Love helps the beloved to become as the lover sees him . . . so he becomes more and more the image of "what God conceived and wanted him to be".[33]

Having described psychotherapy in these terms, Frankl went on to describe various clinical conditions in terms of being and not being responsible for realizing one's inner being. Obsessional neurosis, he indicated, involves the patient replacing true with false responsibility. The melancholic's experience of meaninglessness results from experiencing a hopeless abyss between what is and ought to be. The schizophrenic inauthentically experiences himself as

---

[30] V. Frankl (1965) *The Doctor and the Soul*, New York: Vintage Books, 1973 p. 137.

[31] Ibid. p. 138.

[32] Ibid. p. 149.

[33] Ibid. p. 151.

determined by others, as thing-like object of their intentions and will. It is here that Frankl introduced what I earlier referred to as his "paradoxical intention" method of therapy.[34] It consists of seeking to persuade patients to intend precisely what they most fear.

Examples included a patient crippled by phobic avoidance of situations in which he might sweat. Frankl encouraged him to tell himself whenever he was most frightened of sweating – when he had to shake hands, for instance – "I sweated out only a quart before, but now I'm going to pour out at least ten quarts!".[35] Another example was a 35-year-old woman. Since early childhood she had obsessively spent all her time scrubbing and cleaning. Frankl treated her by inviting her to imitate him rubbing his hands on the floor, telling herself as she did so: "See, I cannot get dirty enough; I can't find enough bacteria!".[36] Other examples included a 17-year-old boy treated for stammering by telling himself to stammer, and a patient terrified of flying lest he have a panic attack treated through being encouraged to become as panicky as he could on the plane. This method of therapy might have been manipulative. But it sought to restore patients to the meaningfulness of exercising their free spirit in choosing and being responsible for their existential being.

Unconscious God

Frankl also put this responsibility in religious terms. In 1975 his 1948 book, *Der unbewusste Gott*, was published in an expanded English version as *The Unconscious God*. It was concerned with what Frankl now called "a religious sense deeply rooted in each and every man's unconscious depths".[37] An example, he said, was one of his students at the US International University in San Diego who said that when he was a psychiatric patient:

> In the darkest moment of my life, when I lay abandoned as an animal in a cage, when because of the forgetfulness induced by ECT I *could not* call out to Him, He was there. In the solitary darkness of the "pit" where men had abandoned me, *He was there*. When I did not know His Name, He was there; God was there.[38]

To this example Frankl added the case of a man who wrote from prison saying how, financially ruined and hopeless, he was visited one day by a court

---

[34] Ibid. p. 220.

[35] Ibid. p. 223.

[36] Ibid. p. 228.

[37] V. Frankl (1975) The Unconscious God, in V. Frankl (2000) *Man's Search of Ultimate Meaning*, New York: Perseus, pp. 1–136, 14.

[38] Ibid. p. 15.

psychiatrist, to whom he took a great liking for indicating, through smiling and shaking his hand, that he was still human – a "somebody". It resulted, that night, in the beginning of his spiritual transformation:

> In the stillness of my small cell, I experienced a most unusual religious feeling which I never had before; I was able to pray, and with utmost sincerity, I accepted a Higher Will to which I have surrendered the pain and sorrow as meaningful and ultimate, not needing explanation. . . . Today, I am at complete peace with myself and the world. I have found the true meaning of my life, and time can only delay its fulfillment but not deter it. At fifty-four, I have decided to reconstruct my life and to finish my schooling.[39]

Such orientation by and through love of another becomes, in religion, wrote Frankl, "man's search for *ultimate* meaning".[40] But love cannot be cajoled or willed. Nor can belief or faith. It is the same with laughter. If you want someone to laugh you must tell him a joke. Similarly, if you want someone to have faith in God you must portray Him believably and act credibly yourself. For religion to survive, said Frankl, it had to become "profoundly personalized".[41]

Again criticizing Freudian psychoanalysis for characterizing us as determined by thing-like instincts and agents – id, ego, and superego – Frankl emphasized the focus of existential analysis on the freedom of the spirit. Unlike psychoanalysis – with its concern to enable people to become conscious of unconscious instincts – he insisted on logotherapy's aim of seeking to enable people to become conscious of their unconscious spirit. Logotherapy is not concerned with the ego becoming conscious of the id, but with the self becoming conscious of itself. The unconscious is not just instinct. It is also spirit. Spirit is the proper object of therapy. Therapy's true aim is to awaken our spirit, freedom, and responsibility against the tendency to regard our fate as determined by instinct. For health and authenticity consist in deciding for ourselves.

The core of our existence is spiritual. In part, therefore, it cannot but be unconscious in so far as our existence cannot be fully reflected upon. It cannot be fully aware of itself. Or, as the Indian Vedas put it, "That which does the seeing, cannot be seen; that which does the hearing cannot be heard; and that which does the thinking, cannot be thought".[42] Similarly that which has to decide whether something is to be conscious or unconscious cannot be conscious.

Saying all this, Frankl added that consciousness should not be confused with conscience. Consciousness is concerned with reality, with what is the case.

---

[39] V. Frankl (1975) The Unconscious God, in V. Frankl (2000) *Man's Search of Ultimate Meaning*, New York: Perseus, pp. 15–16.

[40] Ibid. p. 17.

[41] Ibid. p. 18.

[42] Ibid. p. 37.

Conscience is concerned with possibility, with what ought to be the case. It is concerned with what might be made real. It aims to make real the unique possibilities latent in any life situation. Similarly, Frankl added, love aims at realizing the unique possibilities latent in the beloved. As long as an unconscious instinct determines one's beloved it cannot be love. For, in love, the self is not driven by the id. Rather, in love, "the self chooses the Thou".[43]

It is the same with art. Just as conscience and love are rooted in the intuitive, non-rational depths of the spiritual unconscious, so is art. To illustrate the point, Frankl cited the case of a patient – a violinist – for whom treatment entailed enabling him to trust his unconscious spirit. More generally, Frankl maintained, therapy involves making the unconscious conscious as a means, paradoxically, of enabling consciousness again to become unconscious. Therapy's aim is to soak the self in its unconscious spirit so as to free the patient of the neurotic and psychotic ills resulting from the invasion of consciousness by the unconscious psychological or bodily forces of the id.

We can recover the id through dreams. We can likewise recover our spirit. An example, said Frankl, was a patient who dreamt she went to church, and added:

> When I pass it I often think, I am on the way to God – not through the church directly, but through psychotherapy. My way to God goes, so to speak, through the doctor . . . [In my dream the] church is entirely bombed out; the roof has fallen in, and only the altar remains intact. . . . I find myself on St. Stephen's Square. . . . In the Cathedral it is dark, but I know God is there. . . . I have a box of candy with me, with the inscription on it, "God calls" . . . I am afraid someone may see the inscription on the candy box; I am ashamed and start to erase the inscription.[44]

Like this patient, wrote Frankl, we may avoid our love or orientation to God becoming public in therapy for fear of the therapist erasing or reducing it to a thing. But the spirit of love and religion is not a thing. The spirit is not a thing-like archetype in the unconscious.

Nor is conscience a thing. We can only obey our conscience through having a genuine dialogue with it, through conscience transcending and being other than the self who consults it. It indicates an origin beyond us, just as our navel indicates our origin in someone other than ourselves. Godlessness involves overlooking this transcendent aspect of conscience. The irreligious man is like Samuel in the Old Testament who, wakened in the night by a voice calling his name, did not at first recognize that the voice came from outside him. It took

43 Ibid. p. 42.

44 Ibid. pp. 51–2.

time for him to say, "Speak, Lord; for thy servant heareth".[45] The irreligious man mistakes conscience for fact, just as Freudian psychoanalysis mistakes conscience for an introjected father figure or superego. Reducing conscience to the superego is akin to reducing the self to the ego. Although a function of the self may include repressing and sublimating the drives and instincts, it cannot be derived from them. The drives and instincts cannot be responsible for themselves. Nor can the self be responsible solely to itself. Freudian analysis is therefore mistaken in its fundamental assumption that, as Frankl put it, "the ego pulls itself up by the bootstraps of the superego out of the bog of the id".[46] It overlooks the transcendent character of conscience, the fact that conscience is beyond and other than the self who consults it. Hence, wrote Frankl, his extension of psychoanalysis to include the spirit as well as the psyche.

If we say that the spirit is oriented towards God then, argued Frankl, it is appropriate to speak of an "unconscious God". The Psalms speak of "the hidden God", and Hellenistic culture dedicated an altar to "the unknown God". So too the concept of an unconscious God refers to "man's hidden relation to a God who himself is hidden".[47] But the notion that we have an unconscious orientation to God should not be mistaken to mean that God is within us, and inhabits our unconscious. Nor should it be mistaken to mean that the unconscious is divine, omniscient, and knows the truth better than the conscious self. Nor should we conclude that God is an impersonal force driving us, as Jung implied with his concept of religious archetypes as pre-formed psychological facts within the unconscious making us religious, and choose to take responsibility for ourselves. In this Jung was like Freud, maintained Frankl. Both mistook the unconscious as containing things which drive us.

Frankl then turned to symbols. Contrary to Jung, he argued that they are not born within us. Rather, he maintained, we are born into them. They wait for us to make them our own. This is equally true of religious symbols. Religiousness is not an illusion, as Freud claimed. It is a reality. The task of logotherapy is to enable patients to become conscious of their unconscious religiousness as in the patient whose neurosis results from his repressing his relation to transcendence. Neurosis can be an effect of a crippled relation to transcendence. It is an effect of repressing the angel in us. Or, as Frankl also put it, "once the angel within us is repressed, he turns into a demon".[48]

....

45 V. Frankl (1975) The Unconscious God, in V. Frankl (2000) *Man's Search of Ultimate Meaning*, New York: Perseus, p. 62.

46 Ibid. p. 65.

47 Ibid. p. 68.

48 Ibid. p. 75.

But this does not entail that therapy should become religious indoctrination. Quite the reverse. True religion depends on our freely choosing whether or not to be religious. Religious experience cannot be genuine if we are driven to it by instinct or therapy. It should not be administered like a pill, injection, or electro-shock as means of improving our mental health. Religion may promote our mental health. But this is not its aim. Its aim is not therapy but spiritual salvation.

As long as human existence is not distorted by neurosis it is always freely oriented toward something or someone other than itself. Frankl called this "self-transcendence".[49] This does not entail what the humanistic psychologist, Abe Maslow, called higher and lower needs. Rather it concerns whether our goals are a mere means to an end or a meaningful end in themselves. Rejecting as always Freud's and Adler's focus in analysis on the will to pleasure and power, Frankl insisted that neither constitute a proper end or goal of human existence. Pleasure is not its end. Pleasure is a by-product of self-transcendence. Pursuing happiness for itself is self-defeating. Obvious examples are the neurotic frigidity or impotence of those who pursue sexual pleasure as an end in itself.

Our instincts do not tell us what to do. We can choose. In this we are unlike animals. Nor do we have to do what social tradition tells us to do. Obeying biology or society risks bringing about the existential vacuum of neurosis, conformism, totalitarianism.[50] Unlike animals we can transcend and detach ourselves from ourselves. It was in terms of this capacity for self-detachment that Frankl advocated therapy not only through paradoxical intention but also through behaviour modification.

Advocating these techniques, Frankl maintained that, in seeking to enable its patients find a meaning in their life, logotherapy borrows from what patients know in their unconscious. Logotherapy brings this knowledge to consciousness. An example was a man on death row in San Quentin whom Frankl said he helped by telling him Tolstoy's story about Ivan Ilyich who, realizing "that he has wasted his life, that his life has been virtually meaningless", as Frankl somewhat inaccurately put it, "grows beyond himself and finally becomes capable – retrospectively – of flooding his life with infinite meaning".[51]

Psychology, according to Frankl, only has to resort to drives and instincts if it rules out meaning and self-transcendence. But if life does not reach for anything beyond itself it becomes meaningless. It is not even possible. "This is

49 Ibid. p. 84.

50 Ibid. p. 94.

51 Ibid. p. 129.

the very lesson I learned in three years spent in Auschwitz and Dachau," he wrote at the end of *The Unconscious God*. "Only those who were oriented toward the future, toward a goal in the future, toward a meaning to fulfill in the future, were likely to survive".[52]

World-wide celebrity

Frankl's account of his concentration camp experiences led to his becoming an international celebrity. Even in his nineties he still received letters every day from people telling him his book, *Man's Search for Meaning*, had changed their lives. It certainly changed his life. From the late 1950s onwards he became immensely renowned. Mamie Eisenhower, the widow of the US president, invited him to stay on their estate near Washington. He had a private audience with Pope Paul VI, to whom he spoke of his thanks to God for having given him so many years of life after Auschwitz.[53] He was nominated for a Nobel peace prize. He was given the John F. Kennedy Star, the Albert Schweitzer Medal, and many other awards. He was given honorary degrees by twenty-nine universities across the world. He was appointed to visiting professorships at Harvard, Stanford, Dallas, Pittsburgh, and San Diego. In 1977 an institute of logotherapy, adopting his ideas, was started in Berkeley. Twenty-six similar institutes and societies were subsequently established in the USA and else-where. A community-based home named after him was opened in Hamburg for previously hospitalized psychiatric patients.

Addressing the American Psychiatric Association (APA) Annual Conference in 1985, he reported the finding of another major existential psychotherapist, Irvin Yalom,[54] that a third of his outpatients attributed their problems to meaninglessness. Frankl advocated three ways of achieving meaning: work; love and transcending fate. To illustrate the third way he quoted William James. In a lecture given over a century before, James gave the example of a dog suffering in a vivisection experiment unaware of the good it may do for the future welfare of human and animal life. James contrasted this with the fate of human beings who, however dire their lot, can transcend it through choosing to have faith that it will bear fruit in "an unseen spiritual world" beyond them.[55]

----

[52] V. Frankl (1975) The Unconscious God, in V. Frankl (2000) *Man's Search of Ultimate Meaning*, New York: Perseus, pp. 134–5.

[53] Frankl 1995 p. 124.

[54] I. Yalom (1980) *Existential Psychotherapy*, New York: Perseus.

[55] W. James (1895) Is life worth living? in W. James (1897) *The Will to Believe*, New York: Dover, 1956 pp. 32–62, 58.

Reiterating this example from James, Frankl told the APA that where know-ledge fails faith is needed. An existential decision is required. Belief in God. Belief in being itself. Religion, Frankl went on, is a system of symbols for what we cannot grasp conceptually. When he was 15, he recalled, he had concluded, "God is the partner of our most intimate soliloquies. That is to say, whenever you are talking to yourself in utmost sincerity and ultimate solitude – he to whom you are addressing yourself may justifiably be called God".[56] A religious sense exists in all of us even though it is often buried, repressed, and uncon-scious. Hence even those who are irreligious are just as capable of finding meaning in their lives as those who are religious. Religion fulfills our will to ultimate meaning. As evidence Frankl cited Einstein talking of being religious giving life sense, and Wittgenstein saying "To believe in God is to see that life has a meaning".[57]

The same year, 1995, as Frankl gave this lecture he was made an honorary citizen of Vienna. He continued to live there but he had heart problems, and on 2 September 1997 he died. By then he was such a celebrity the Austrian Chancellor, Viktor Klima, gave a speech in his memory. He lauded him as a "great humanist, scientist, and world citizen".[58] He remains a celebrity. His work lives on. It is still very popular, in large part because of his faith – despite or because of his concentration camp experiences – in the inherent goodness and free spirit of human existence. In this, however, he was rather like the mind-cure and other religious therapists whom William James called the "once-born" and criticized as over-optimistically believing in goodness to the neglect of what is bad. This brings me to Melanie Klein, who certainly did not forget badness, as I will now relate.

---

56 V. Frankl (1995) Man's search for ultimate meaning, in V. Frankl (2000) *Man's Search for Ultimate Meaning*, Cambridge, Massachusetts: Perseus, pp. 137–54, 151.

57 Ibid. p. 153.

58 R. Prinz (1997) Viktor E. Frankl, at 92; noted psychiatrist, author, *Bergen Record Corp.*, www.bergen.com/obits/obfrankl.htm.

Chapter 8

Melanie Klein

Healing grace

Melanie Klein's version of psychoanalysis and religion is not nearly so popular as that of Viktor Frankl. There is much to dislike about her work. Particularly odious and questionable – both factually and therapeutically – is her emphasis on hate, envy, and badness as effect of an instinct toward death and destruction existing innately and independently of an instinct for love, goodness, and life with which she believed we are also born.

Nevertheless, despite her emphasis on hate, Klein's approach to therapy is also very promising in emphasizing, as did William James, transformation from self-division between good and bad into wholeness and health through the grace of recognizing and feeling gratitude and love for what is good. However, whereas James described this transformation in religious terms, Klein described it entirely secularly. Unlike Jung, Fromm, Tillich, and Frankl, she did not ally religion and psychoanalysis. Like Freud, she almost entirely rejected religion in favour of single-minded pursuit of psychoanalysis.

Religious ambivalence

Perhaps it would be more accurate to say that just as Klein later emphasized our ambivalence – our love and hate – she was also ambivalent about religion. She was born in Vienna on 30 March 1882 to Jewish parents – Moriz and Libussa Reizes – who already had three children. Melanie was their youngest child. She later described her early upbringing as "anti-Orthodox".[1] Nevertheless the family kept Friday evening prayers, the Passover meal, and fasted on the Day of Atonement. Her mother, Libussa, also tried to keep a kosher kitchen till the children rebelled. And Melanie envied and even one day copied the Catholic children at school running up to kiss the priest's hand to be patted by him.

Through her older brother, Emmanuel, Melanie became involved in Vienna's cultural and university life, but she never completed a degree. When she was 17

---

[1] In P. Grosskurth (1986) *Melanie Klein*, London: Hodder & Stoughton, p. 13.

she became engaged to a cousin, Arthur Klein, a chemical engineer from Zurich who, despite being Jewish, had been sent to a Jesuit school before going to university. They married on 31 March 1903 and, in 1910, settled near Arthur's Catholic sister and her family in Budapest, where Arthur and Melanie joined the Unitarian church. All three of their children were also baptized.[2]

Settled in Budapest, Melanie read Freud's 1901 book, *On Dreams*. Having suffered with depression after becoming a mother, she also went into analysis – with Ferenczi. Encouraged by his experiments in child analysis, she analysed her youngest child, Erich. In reporting his treatment, as though it were that of another child, Fritz, she described herself, as his mother, as an atheist who nevertheless did not repudiate the ready-made version of God taught her children by others. She also mentioned how, when Erich was four and asked her, "Does God know for certain how long he will let it rain?", she replied evasively by saying God does not make the rain, it comes from the clouds. She was similarly evasive when he asked her the next day whether God was real. She simply said she had never seen him. But, when Erich again asked, she was more explicit. She told him, "No, child, he is not real".[3] When he again asked her about God that evening, she said, "I have never seen him and do not believe either that God exists", to which his father added, "some people believe that God exists and others believe that he doesn't. I believe that he does but your mamma believes that he doesn't". At this Erich declared, "I think too that there is no God".[4] Through admitting their disagreement, Klein concluded, she and her husband freed their son to think for himself. More generally, she argued, since the idea of God can be so inhibiting to discovering what is true, children are better off without it.

Klein recounted her analysis of Erich to a psychoanalytic congress held in Budapest in July 1919. Soon after this a violently anti-semitic counter-revolution, following Hungary's previous Bolshevik uprising, led to Arthur losing his job and going to work in Sweden. Meanwhile Melanie went with the children to live with his parents in Rosenberg from where, after going to a psychoanalytic congress in The Hague where Abraham invited her to join his psychoanalytic centre in Berlin, she moved there with Erich in January 1921.

Child analysis

Melanie Klein now began analysing children other than her own. She used their play, as Freud used his patients' dreams, to access their unconscious.

---

[2] Klein's children were Melitta (born on 19 January 1904), Hans (born on 2 March 1907), and Erich (born on 6 November 1914).

[3] M. Klein (1921) The development of a child, **WMK1** pp. 1–53, 6.

[4] Ibid. p. 7.

Addressing the hatred as well as love they transferred from their parents into their play with her, Klein became convinced that the source of children's psychological difficulties often lies in hating their parents' love-making. An example was a 3-year-old, Peter, whose difficulties she traced to his witnessing his parents making love when he was eighteen months old. In his first therapy session with her, he arguably represented this by putting some toy carriages and cars behind each other. He then put them side by side, knocked two toy horses together, and said, "And now they are going to sleep". He then buried them with bricks, saying "Now they're quite dead". Another time he put two pencils together on a sponge and shouted at them in a voice like that of his father. He castigated them as he perhaps also wanted to castigate his parents making love, telling them, "You're not to go about together all the time and do piggish things".[5]

But this gave rise to a fearful image of his father taking revenge on him. More often, however, Klein discovered that children are less fearful of their fathers than of their mothers, at least at first. An example was a 4-year-old patient, Ruth, who, transferred her fear of her mother onto Klein as her analyst. Initially Ruth was so frightened of Klein that her older sister had to accompany her when she came for analysis. One day she rummaged in her sister's bag and then shut it tight, "so that nothing should fall out", she explained. She did the same with her sister's purse. Then she drew a tumbler with balls inside it and a lid on top – "to prevent the ball from rolling out". It was the same with her mother. She wanted to keep her babies safely shut up inside her, to stop them coming out and upsetting her as she had been upset by her mother giving birth to her younger sister.

Another time she played at giving dolls jugfuls of milk to drink. But when Klein put a wet sponge near one of them, Ruth insisted, "No, she mustn't have the big sponge, that's not for children, that's for grown-ups!" She could not bear to have what her mother had in making love with her father. The sponge, said Klein, represented his penis inside her. It made Ruth want to get into her mother and attack, harm, and rob her of the goodness and love inside her. But this led her to imagine that her mother might similarly attack her. It also led to her transferring onto Klein this fear based on hatred of love.

Klein argued that children's resulting "phantasies" (as she spelt "fantasy" to emphasize its unconscious origin)[6] stem from children feeling deprived of love – at least of their mother's milk and of their faeces – on being weaned and

---

[5] M. Klein (1932) *The Psycho-Analysis of Children*, **WMK2** pp. 17, 23.

[6] See e.g. E. Bott Spillius (2001) Freud and Klein on the concept of phantasy, *IJPA*, **82** pp. 361–73.

potty-trained by her. Examples of children hating and attacking their mothers included a 3-year-old patient, Trude. In therapy with Klein, she pretended it was night and that they were both asleep. She then came over to Klein, threatened to hit her in the stomach, take out her faeces, and make her poor. At this Trude became terrified, hid behind the sofa, covered herself, sucked her fingers, and wet herself. She thereby re-enacted, it seemed, a scenario in which, when she was not quite two, she would run into her parents' bedroom at night as though wanting to rob her pregnant mother of her baby. But this made her fearful lest her mother – and Klein in her analysis – similarly attack her. It was this, said Klein, that led to the night-time terrors for which she had originally been referred for analysis.

Klein presented some of these findings to the psychoanalytic congress held in Salzburg in April 1924. That autumn, at a psychoanalytic congress in Würzburg, she spoke more about children hating their parents' love-making, and about their fantasies. She talked about an only child, a 6-year-old, Erna, whose symptoms – obsessive head-banging, rocking, thumb-sucking, and compulsive masturbating – seemingly began after a family holiday when she was two, shared her parents' bedroom, and saw them "wiggle-woggling" together.[7]

In analysis she cast Klein in the role of the mother cruelly excluding her from the oral, anal, and genital pleasures she imagined her mother enjoying in making love with her father. She got Klein to suck an engine with gilded lamps – "all red and burning" – just as she arguably imagined her mother enjoying sucking her father's penis. Then, taking the place of her mother, Erna sucked the lamps herself. She also sucked her thumb. Other times she played at "wurling" fish with a policeman father, while Klein had to look on as the excluded child trying to get in and take the fish from them. Or she pretended to dirty herself, incited Klein to scold her, and then retaliated by vomiting up bad food, whereupon she became anxious lest Klein similarly attack her. She talked of a flea, all "black and yellow mixed", like a piece of food or shit, coming out of Klein's body, attacking and forcing itself into her. Putting these fantasies into words, said Klein, enabled Erna to distinguish more clearly between her actual mother and her fantasies about her. As a result her image of her mother, and her play, became more tender and loving as she felt less driven to ward off hateful feelings and fantasies of deprivation with the symptoms bringing her into treatment.

---

[7] Klein 1932 p. 49 n. 2.

Whatever the success of her treatment, Erna's hateful talk of making her parents into "mincemeat" and "eye-salad" hardly endeared Klein's Berlin colleagues to her. They denounced her work as embarrassing and ridiculous. They said she was "feeble-minded about theory".[8] Psychoanalytic colleagues in Vienna were similarly critical when she spoke to them about her work in December 1924. Psychoanalysts in London, however, proved more sympathetic when James Strachey gave an account of her work to the British Psycho-Analytical Society (BPAS) in January 1925. As a result she was invited to talk about her work in London that July. Her return to Berlin, however, was bleak. A love affair, begun that spring, ended and on Christmas day, her analyst, Karl Abraham, suddenly died leaving her with nobody to defend her against her Berlin psychoanalyst critics. She therefore gladly accepted an invitation from Ernest Jones, then President of the BPAS, to analyse his children. She returned to London in September 1926 and lived first in a flat in the Temple, and then in a maisonette near the Institute of Psycho-Analysis in Gloucester Place. Finally she settled in Notting Hill from where her son, Erich, attended St Paul's School.

Meanwhile, in Vienna, Freud's psychoanalyst daughter, Anna, criticized Klein's approach to child analysis. She argued that children are too closely involved with their parents to entertain fantasies of love and hate about them. To illustrate her contrary claim, Klein recounted the case of a 4-year-old who, despite his parents apparently loving and never punishing or threatening him, nevertheless had fantasies about them hatefully eating him up, cutting him to pieces, and castrating him. These fantasies, claimed Klein, were evident in his variously imagining her as an ideally lovable fairy godmother and as a hatefully wicked witch. Enabling children to play, enabling their minds to develop, she argued, depends on putting their negative (as well as their positive) fantasies into words rather than reinforcing them by advocating, like Anna Freud, that child analysis should strengthen children's image of their parents and psychoanalysts as superego authority figures within them.

Klein summarized the findings of her quite different approach to analysis in a talk she gave to a meeting of psychoanalysts held in Innsbruck in September 1927. In her talk she maintained that the first object of children's fantasies is the mother. She accordingly characterized children's initial development as going through a "femininity phase".[9] Subsequently, she said, the sexes diverge.

---

[8] To James from Alix Strachey, Berlin, 11 January 1925, in P. Meisel and W. Kendrick (1986) *Bloomsbury/Freud*, London: Chatto & Windus, p. 180.

[9] M. Klein (1928) Early stages of the Oedipus conflict, **WMK1** pp. 186–98, 189.

The boy fends off fear of his mother, as a hatefully attacking figure within him, by reassuring himself that, whatever his mother's hateful attack on him, his penis remains intact. Girls, by contrast, lack any such outward reassurance.

To further illustrate children's fantasies of love and hate, Klein recounted the libretto by Colette for Maurice Ravel's opera, *L'enfant et les sortilèges*. It begins with a little boy not wanting to do his homework. He would much rather go to the park, pull the cat's tail and scold everyone, particularly his mother. When she comes in and asks if he has finished his homework, he puts his tongue out at her, whereupon she punishes him saying, "You shall have dry bread and no sugar in your tea".[10] At this he flies into a rage, attacks the tea things, the pets, the fire and the pendulum inside a grandfather clock – just as the Oedipal child, said Klein, seeks to attack his father's penis inside his mother in their love-making. But then everything comes vengefully alive. A wild rumpus starts. The little boy tries to find refuge in the park. But he is attacked there too. Animals fight and bite him. Concerned about a squirrel who falls to the ground, the boy picks it up and binds its injured paw. With this everything is transformed. Everything becomes more loving, appreciated, and friendly: "He is restored to the human world of helping, 'being good'."[11]

Klein also recounted an extreme example of love obstructed by hate in the case of an autistic 4-year-old, Dick. As a baby, it seems, Dick had been so over-whelmed by dread of his own aggression and hatred in sucking and feeding he scarcely did either. He nearly died of starvation. He was also seemingly starved of love by his mother and wet-nurse. With the loving care of another nurse and his grandmother, however, he survived, became toilet-trained, and learnt a few words. But he still refused to eat anything but pre-mashed food. Nor was he interested in anything except doors, door handles, and trains. Klein under-stood this in terms of children's fantasies about getting into their mothers as they imagine their fathers doing in making love. She tried to engage Dick's interest by taking up two trains. She called one "Daddy", the other "Dick". At this Dick took up the "Dick" train and rolled it to the window saying "Station" whereupon Klein commented, "The station is Mummy: Dick is going into Mummy". With this he became fearful and ran into the dark space between the inner and outer doors of her room. This happened again in their subsequent meetings together. He became increasingly emotionally involved, and aware not only of fear for himself, but also of love and concern for Klein. One day, for instance, having scratched a toy coal-cart, thrown it into a drawer and

---

[10] M. Klein (1929) Infantile anxiety situations reflected in a work of art and in the creative impulse, ibid. pp. 210–18, 210.

[11] Ibid. p. 211.

covered it with the other toys, he put them all into her lap, saying sadly "Poor Mrs Klein".[12] Klein followed up her account of his treatment by announcing, in 1935, her theory of what she called "the depressive position".

Depressive position

In announcing this theory, Klein again emphasized hate as well as love. She argued that both impulses are present from the beginning of life, that new-born babies imagine their mothers as both all-loving and all-hating. They also entertain fantasies, she said, of getting into the mother, and of scooping out, devouring, and destroying everything inside her. But, said Klein, the baby also increasingly loves the mother – in the first place her breast – as whole, intact, and good.

Loving the mother as a good figure inside themselves enables babies to countenance also experiencing her as hated and bad. They no longer feel so driven to divide one image from the other. But, in becoming less self-divided through the transforming and integrating effect of love, babies become fearful, said Klein, that, in attacking the mother they hate, they might lose the mother they love. For they now realize the two mothers are one and the same. They also feel guilty and concerned lest hatred damage, ruin, or even kill their mothers. This impels the baby to try to put the damage right – to revive, repair and restore his mother.

But babies, children, and adults can also feel overwhelmed by the work of repairing the damage done by their hatred and destruction. They may defend against recognizing this damage, and against awareness of their love of others, with self-preoccupied hypochondria and persecutory fear for themselves. Or, they may defend with manic denial of dependence on others, and with denial of their inner feelings – including their ambivalence – and instead indulge fantasies of omnipotence, control, and contempt.

It was this constellation of fearing losing those we love through hate, and the manic and other defences this evokes, that Klein called "the depressive position".[13] She described it as evoked whenever we experience loss of, or threatened loss of those we love. She illustrated the point by recounting, as though it were the experience of one of her patients, her reaction to her son, Hans, being killed in a mountain accident in April 1934. At first, following his

---

[12] M. Klein (1930) The importance of symbol-formation in the development of the ego, ibid. pp. 219–32, 227.

[13] M. Klein (1935) A contribution to the psychogenesis of manic-depressive states, ibid. pp. 262–89, 271.

death, she idealized him. She kept everything she felt was good of his and threw out everything she felt was bad. She also dreamt that it was not him but her brother, Emmanuel, who had died. She felt hostile to both him and her mother, whom she also felt she controlled and triumphed over in her dream. This was followed by more loving feelings. She took comfort in looking at pleasantly situated houses in the country. She thought she would like to have one herself. She began to trust in the existence of good, loving, and loved people. As a result, she said, she felt less driven to control others in her mind. She was thereby able both to grieve and recover her love of her son through these inner figures becoming more alive as comforting and grieving with her in her loss.

Another example, this time from her psychoanalytic work rather than from her self-analysis, involved a man who, the night before his mother died, dreamt he was with her, that a dangerous bull was between them, and that he fled leaving her unprotected. It reminded him of shooting buffalo to eat and of buffalo being an endangered species, needing protection. He arrived at his next analytic session hating Klein. Unconsciously, it seems, he equated her with his dream of his mother with the bull, representing his father. Only when Klein reminded him of this image's counterpart – the buffalo needing protection – did he acknowledge and tell her of his mother's death. Klein's reminder, it seems, also enabled him to be more generally conscious of love and concern for protecting the well-being of others, and he less often saw his "dear old parents",[14] as he called them, as the attacking and attacked figures which had previously thwarted his love for them and others.

Klein also illustrated the implications for therapy of her theory of the depressive position with the example of a 10-year-old, Richard, whom she began treating in April 1941. His symptoms included being so fearful of others he had not been able to go to school since he was 8, and fear of the war, not least because his home had been bombed. Through Klein putting into words the depressive position expression and cause, in her view, of his symptoms in fear of loss of love, and defence against the work of repairing it, Richard became calmer, more trusting and hopeful of Klein and others. He experienced the room in which they met as cosier. He drew pictures in which his image of his mother became friendlier and more loving. He began recalling good early memories. And he sought to keep Klein as a good figure in his mind, or so Klein wrote, by having her help him tie his shoelaces, by thinking of becoming an analyst like her, and by taking a photograph of her. It enabled him to become more confident, she wrote, of being able to end his analysis and go back to school.

---

[14] M. Klein (1940) Mourning and its relation to manic-depressive states, ibid. pp. 344–69, 368.

With her theory of the depressive position (transforming of self-division through gratitude and love) rather than the Oedipus complex as central turning point in our psychology, Klein alienated many psychoanalysts. They were particulary critical of her theory that children very early on experience goodness and love, as well as badness and hate, of those around them as internal figures or objects within their minds. Conflict between her supporters and detractors nearly tore the BPAS apart during the war. The BPAS, however, was saved by its members agreeing to disagree. With the future of her work assured, Klein now put forward the theory that the depressive position is preceded by what she called "the paranoid–schizoid position".

Paranoid–schizoid position

Klein first presented this theory to the BPAS on 4 December 1946. In doing so she approvingly cited the paediatrician and psychoanalyst Donald Winnicott's account, the previous year, of what she called "the unintegration of the early ego".[15] She attributed this unintegration to an effect of an inborn death instinct which, she said, expresses itself in the baby's fear of "falling to pieces".[16] Splitting off, and projecting this destructive effect of the "death instinct" into the mother, the baby also wards off anxiety by introjecting her as a "good object".[17] In doing so, he may omnipotently idealize her, or her breast, as "inexhaustible and always bountiful".[18] This, in turn, may evoke hateful impulses of greedily robbing her of what is loved and good inside her, and of enviously expelling spoiling hatred into her. This entails what Klein now called "projective identification".[19]

Projective identification, she said, involves identifying with someone else – in the first place with the mother – through projecting into them hated parts of oneself such that one may then feel persecuted by them. Or one can identify with others through projecting and identifying with loved parts of oneself in them with the result that one might feel impoverished and empty in oneself. An example, said Klein, was a patient who denuded herself of good parts of herself by projecting them into, and becoming preoccupied with Greta Garbo as standing for herself. Another example, said Klein, is the character, Fabian, in

---

[15] M. Klein (1946) Notes on some schizoid mechanisms, **WMK3** pp. 1–24, 4.

[16] Ibid. p. 5.

[17] Ibid. p. 6.

[18] Ibid. p. 7.

[19] Ibid. p. 8.

a novel by Julian Green, who escapes his life as a petty official, made dreary by lack of love, by making a pact with the devil enabling him to get into and become others so as to enjoy, albeit in alienated form, the goodness and love he projects and envies in them.

Klein described this second example in a chapter of a book published in 1955.[20] At that year's psychoanalytic congress in Geneva she spoke more about envy. She spoke about how life instinct-based love of what is good in others may paradoxically give rise to its opposite – death instinct-based hatred. This may include hate-driven greedy expropriation, and envious spoiling of what is loved as good in others. An example, she said, was a patient who rubbished her as unlovable and no good. The patient dreamt Klein was a contemptible, apathetic, and useless cow on whom the patient scornfully looked down from a magic carpet, whilst Klein, as the cow, munched an endless strip of blanket, as though eating her interpretations as woolly and worthless. By explaining how the patient thereby sought enviously to spoil the understanding she wanted, Klein claimed, she helped her counter her destructive envy of the goodness she wanted so as to become conscious of, and experience analysis as beneficial and good.

Klein said more about envy and destruction of what is loved and good, and about its counterpart, gratitude for what is recognized as loved and good, in a talk in May 1959 to a group of sociologists in which, unusually for her, she spoke favourably about religion:

> It is not for nothing that in saying grace before meals, Christians use the words, "For what we are about to receive may the Lord make us truly thankful". These words imply that one asks for the one quality – gratitude – which will make one happy and free from resentment and envy.[21]

In another talk that summer, 1959, she dwelt on loneliness. She linked it to our first longing for the love and understanding of our mothers as babies. Loneliness, she said, arises from longing to recover love lost through projecting it into others, or through destroying it with envious or greedy hatred. A case in point, she said, was a man who sought to counteract his loneliness with love of the country only to find it ruined by childhood memories of greedily robbing birds' nests and enviously damaging hedges. If only, he yearned, he could grow things all might be well.

Klein herself became very unwell the next year on holiday in Switzerland. She was brought back to London and after having an operation for cancer,

---

[20] M. Klein (1955) On identification, ibid. pp. 141–75.

[21] M. Klein (1959) Our adult world and its roots in infancy, ibid. pp. 247–63, 254.

died that autumn, on 22 September 1960. Among her papers were found the following notes about religion:

> Christ as the good part of God. The harsh and persecuting God was so much mitigated by having a son who is the representative of love and forgiveness but who forms part of him. Christ said "I am in my father and my father is in me"; it may have been unbearable to have this lonely and harsh punishing God who was an internalised figure and therefore increased their own super-ego and anxieties . . . in heaven there is to be no hate, only love – finding again relatives with whom there had been envy hate jealousy – where will be wholesale reparation because only love – religion an expression of life instinct.[22]

More enduring – for psychoanalysis and psychotherapy – Klein left writings indicating ways in which the fragmentation of paranoid–schizoid self-division might be transformed through grace, gratitude, and love into depressive position wholeness, reparation, and creativity. In this she often emphasized inner rather than outer reality. Healing through goodness in outer nature and art is much better brought out by her follower, the art critic, Adrian Stokes, with whose work I will accordingly end this chapter.

Healing goodness: Adrian Stokes

Like Melanie Klein (with whom he was in analysis from 1929 to 1936 and then again briefly in 1938 and 1946),[23] Stokes did not believe in God. Drawing on her theory of the integration achieved by internalizing what is loved and good within us, he said:

> The only way to do without religion is to welcome and foster the original sense of interior goodness . . . since we harbour the idea of a good object (i.e. God) . . . it is a contradiction to conceive this power to be also outside us. Indeed, the essence of the fantasy is that the good object lives at the root of our imagination rather than in Nature, the universe, the outside world.[24]

Freud, as we have seen, criticized Jung's account of the inwardness of schizophrenia as involving heightened interest in the divine. In doing so, Freud emphasized that mental health resides not in inward withdrawal but in engaging with outer reality. To this Adrian Stokes added that outwardness is not only the criterion of health. It also heals inward disorder. Shortly after the final ending of his analysis with Klein, he recalled a moment of Pauline

---

[22] In Grosskurth pp. 454–5.

[23] R. Read (2002) *Art and its Discontents: The Early Life of Adrian Stokes*, Abingdon: Ashgate.

[24] A. Stokes (1945) *Venice*, **CW2** pp. 85–138, 135, 136.

conversion, as it were, in terms of himself, aged 19, going by train from the dark of northern Europe, through the Cenis railway tunnel into the light of Italy:

> The sun shone, the sky was a deep, deep, bold blue . . . the pure note of the guard's horn . . . sustained and reinforced the process by which time was here laid out as ever-present space . . . a revealing of things . . . happening entirely outside me . . . [so that] I could not then fear . . . for what might be hidden inside.[25]

He described particularly well the allaying of inner fear and formlessness through what is outward in a talk he gave to the Imago Society, founded in 1954 to discuss applications of psychoanalysis beyond therapy. He began his resulting essay, "Form in art", with the projection of what is inward outwards. "I find in the clouds today", he wrote, "the splendid shapes of T'ang figures". Art, he went on, does the same. It "projects emotional stress". It transforms inner stress into outer form, into "an entity", into "a world of its own . . . as if the various emotions had been rounded like a stone . . . homogeneity or fusion combined, in differing proportions, with the sense of object-otherness".[26] He described art's transforming effect, as Freud described mystical religious experience, as "oceanic". To this he added, "Because it combines the sense of fusion with the sense of object-otherness, we might say that art is an emblem of the state of being in love".[27]

Art bears witness, said Stokes, to "chaos overcome".[28] But if, as Kleinian analysis suggests, oneness with another is a regressive, omnipotent, or projective identification defence, how can it be a source of health? Stokes asked "How can it be that the homogeneity associated with idealization (the inexhaustible breast), is harnessed by the work of art to an acute sense of otherness and of actuality?"[29]

The answer, he wrote, lies in "just proportion" of fusion and object-otherness making "their harmony poignant and health-giving".[30] In his support he quoted Marion Milner, who, writing about her work as a psychoanalyst, speculated that regression to "states of oneness are perhaps a recurrently necessary

----

25 A. Stokes (1947) *Inside Out*, ibid. pp. 139–82, 156, 157.

26 A. Stokes (1955) Form in art, in M. Klein, P. Heimann and R. Money-Kyrle (eds) *New Directions in Psycho-Analysis*, London: Hogarth, pp. 406–20, 406, 407.

27 Ibid. p. 407.

28 Ibid. p. 413 cf. Apollinaire saying of Matisse, "To make order out of chaos – that is creation", *La Phalange*, 15 December 1970, in *Apollinaire on Art*, London: Thames & Hudson, 1972, pp. 36–9, 38.

29 A. Stokes (1955) p. 414.

30 Ibid. p. 415.

phase in the continued growth of the sense of two-ness" without which it would be impossible "to find new objects, to find the familiar in the unfamiliar".[31] Indeed healthful oneness in two-ness is implicit in Klein's assertion, said Stokes, that:

> The introjection of the good object, first of all the mother's breast, is a precondition of normal development . . . a focal point in the ego. It counteracts the processes of splitting and dispersal, makes for cohesiveness and integration, and is instrumental in building up the ego.[32]

Stokes illustrated all this in terms of the sculpture and poetry of the Christian Platonist, Michelangelo. Writing about him, Stokes again reiterated his thesis that art "offers us some share in the oceanic feeling and at the same time the lover's recognition of his or her beloved's 'singularity' and 'otherness' ".[33] He also reiterated Klein's notion of the integrating, transforming, and creative effect of internalizing those we love within us. He noted how, following the death of one of his brothers, Michelangelo wrote, as if to his dead father, "My brother is painted on my memory but you, father, are sculpted alive in the middle of my heart".[34] Stokes went on to describe this as the transforming source of Michelangelo's art. An example, he wrote, was Michelangelo's *Pietà* in Florence Cathedral:

> He [the father] supports the right arm of the dead Christ and seems to be turning the corpse even more to the side of the Virgin who has Christ's head upon her cheek. We see Michelangelo, then, the most unaccustomed figure, in the exotic paternal role (more active than is St Joseph as a rule) of consigning the son to his mother . . . . deeply moving because, in a reversed form, we are able to partake, as was the artist in carving it, of an ideal reconciliation.[35]

Having thus written about Michelangelo, Stokes turned to Plato and his notion of goodness. Plato emphasized that what he called the Form of the Good – which Christian Platonists, like Simone Weil, equate with God – lies outside us. Just as Klein later argued that love of goodness is inborn, so too, in a sense, did Plato. He quoted Socrates, insisting:

> Before we began to see and hear and use our other senses we must somewhere have acquired the knowledge that there is absolute equality . . . [this] applies [likewise] . . . to absolute beauty, goodness, uprightness, holiness . . . we must have

---

[31] A. Stokes (1955) pp. 417, 418.

[32] Ibid. p. 418, see also Klein 1946 p. 6.

[33] A. Stokes (1955) *Michelangelo*, in **CW3** pp. 7–76, 10, 11.

[34] Ibid. p. 27.

[35] Ibid. p. 49.

obtained knowledge of all these characteristics before our birth . . . afterwards by the exercise of our senses upon sensible objects, [we] recover the knowledge which we had once before.[36]

Plato likened goodness to the sun:

> The Good has begotten it in its own likeness, and it bears the same relation to sight and visibility in the visible world that the Good bears to intelligence and intelligibility in the intelligible world.[37]

Turning towards the good entails turning away from flux – "from the world of change until it [the mind] can bear to look straight at reality, and at the brightest of all realities which is what we call the Good".[38] It entails having an ordered personality, its three aspects – understanding, enterprising spirit, and desire – all in harmony.[39]

Stokes put this in Kleinian terms. He argued that the ordered personality advocated by Plato is achieved through loving, introjecting, and identifying with what is good – in the first place with the mother's breast – to constitute what Stokes, following Klein, called "the core of an integrated ego".[40] Quoting Klein, he said it involves "being alive, loving, and being loved by the internal and external good object".[41] He emphasized the healing effect of being enveloped by what is whole and good in art which, in the visual arts, is necessarily outside and contemplated from a distance. Art, he argued, particularly obviously so in Cubism, also breaks up what it portrays and at the same time brings the fragments together. In doing so it makes them bearable, like the binding – "*religio*", in Latin – of religion.[42]

In thus bringing together psychoanalysis with religion, Adrian Stokes drew on Klein's theories of the transformation wrought by grace – by recognition of, and gratitude for what is good through depressive position integration of the fragmentation of paranoid–schizoid states of mind. Stokes, as I have said, also went beyond Klein in emphasizing the healing effect of oneness with outside object-otherness. It was left to others, however, notably to Marion Milner, to relate this in more detail to religion – specifically to mysticism – and to therapy.

....

[36] Plato (n.d.) *Phaedo*, in *The Last Days of Socrates*, Harmondsworth: Penguin, 1954, pp. 97–183, 124, 125. See also p. 93 above.

[37] Plato (n.d.) *The Republic*, Harmondsworth: Penguin, 1955, p. 272.

[38] Ibid. p. 283.

[39] Ibid. p. 355.

[40] A. Stokes (1958) *Greek Culture and the Ego*, **CW3** pp. 77–141, 86.

[41] Ibid. p. 97.

[42] Ibid. p. 121.

Chapter 9

Marion Milner

Recovering mysticism

Freud, Klein, and other psychoanalysts, both in the past and today, diagnose the experience of oneness with another involved in religious experience as evidence of mental ill-health. They variously diagnose it as a defensive retreat to infantile primary narcissism, manic grandiosity, melancholic fusion with another, or paranoid–schizoid projective identification. Many others, however, psychoanalysts included, emphasize that, as well as being a source of ill-health, recovering our earliest sense of oneness with another is also crucial to our being psychologically alive, creative and well. Marion Milner related this to religious or mystical experience. On first reading her, I have to admit, I balked at her writing which seemed to be overly whimsical, inward, and sensuously self-preoccupied. Re-reading and reading more of what she has to say, I find myself increasingly attracted to her account of mysticism and psychoanalysis and I will try to convey some of its appeal in this chapter. I will begin, however, not with her inward-looking mysticism but with her early outwardly-oriented interest in nature and science.

Outwardly-oriented science

Marion's family included at least two major inventors or scientists. One of her forebears, Charles Babbage, invented the first prototype computer or calculating machine. Her brother, Patrick Blackett, born on 18 November 1897, became a Nobel prize winner for his discoveries in nuclear physics. Marion herself was born on 1 February 1900. Together with Patrick and her older sister, Winifred, she was brought up in Guildford, from where their father, Arthur, travelled to work in the Stock Exchange in London. His father was a parson, and Marion later remembered Arthur himself as "a dreamy Victorian romantic".[1] He loved birdwatching, fishing and poetry. They used to take their holidays in a castle on the Northumberland coast, and Marion later remembered

---

[1] From an interview with Marion Milner on 30 September 1988, in J. Sayers (1989) *Marion Milner, B. P. S. Psychology of Women Newsletter*, no. 3 (Spring), pp. 3–13, 3.

from this time her father walking all night, taking a copy of Shakespeare with him.

When Marion was 11 he had a schizophrenic breakdown. It embittered her against her family's Church of England religion, which failed to cure him with its ritual of "laying on of hands".[2] His breakdown, she said, made her want to look outwards:

> It made me want to be clear about facts. I decided I wanted to become a naturalist – I read that they kept notes. So I started keeping a nature diary, including drawings and paintings of my own. It lasted ten years. At Guilford High School my report (in 1914) said I needed the mental training of Maths and Latin – but learning physiology at the university taught me much more mental training – the difference between facts and theories.[3]

She filled her nature diaries with fresh, delicate, and precise water colour sketches of downland and seashore life, together with details of the nesting and mating habits of the animals in the country near where they lived. They contained nothing about her inner world,[4] about her emotions which, she later said, included feeling confused, abandoned, and intensely angry at her parents going away together for a month, during her father's convalescence, leaving her and her brother and sister with a distant relative. She became severely ill with whooping cough and flu, suffered ear abscesses, and was kept off school for a term because she was thought to be working too hard.

Like her father, however, she also had an air of dreaminess about her. A wealthy aunt bequeathed the family money because, she said, Marion and her sister seemed "not worldly".[5] The money enabled the family to move to Hindhead where their father, feeling a failure, became a postman. Perhaps it also helped pay for Marion to board at Godolphin School in the summer of 1915. From that time she later recalled "sitting at French lessons gazing through the window at the dim line of woods that cloaked the Downs, so deeply longing to be there that my whole body ached with it".[6] Soon, it seems, she was also enjoying mysticism and, when she was 17, she was awarded the *Oxford Book of Mystic Pictures* as a school prize.

----

2 N. R. Dragstedt (1998) Creative illusions: The theoretical and clinical work of Marion Milner (1900–1998), *Journal of Melanie Klein and Object Relations*, **16**(3) pp. 425–536, 436.

3 In Sayers 1989 p. 3.

4 M. Walters (2000) Marion Milner: On Robinson Crusoe's Island, Marion Milner Centenary Conference, Squiggle Foundation, London, 5 February.

5 Dragstedt p. 436.

6 J. Field (1937) *An Experiment in Leisure*, London: Virago, 1986, p. 9.

Not wanting to stay on at school to study for university entrance, she left and earned money teaching a 7-year-old to read. After lessons, she took him to the nearby heath to catch newts and, wanting to learn more about teaching through following children's own interests, she went to the Montessori nursery school training college in Gypsy Hill. From there she went to University College London where she studied psychology and physiology. She was much more interested then, she said, in the body than in the mind, in the big rather than "little sagacity", as Nietzsche put it.[7] Accordingly she was not immediately drawn to Freud when her brother gave her Freud's newly translated *Introductory Lectures on Psycho-Analysis*.

In 1923 she graduated with a first class degree, and went on to do scientific research and vocational guidance work with the National Institute of Industrial Psychology (NIIP). Feeling there must be more to life than collecting facts, however, she pursued a mental training course described in a book her brother gave her. Together with reading Montaigne's *Essays* emphasizing that the soul is quite different from what one might expect, the course led her to begin writing a diary of her self-analysis. She now also came across an article by Elton Mayo contrasting daydreaming reverie and deliberately directed thought. To learn more about his findings she went with her husband, Dennis Milner, whom she had married earlier that year (1927) to Boston to study with Mayo. Whilst in Boston she also went into three times a week therapy with a Jungian analyst, and continued in therapy, with her husband, on their return, in 1929, to London. They bought a house near Chalk Farm and in 1932 Marion gave birth to their only child, John. Soon after the first of several books describing her experiments with mysticism was published under a pseudonym, Joanna Field.

First experiments in mysticism

William James, as we have seen, described mystical experience as ineffable (beyond words), noetic (insightful), transient, and passive. These characteristics, particularly passive surrender, were central to Marion's account of the discoveries she made through her experiments with mysticism. She began her first book about them with Descartes who, following a mystical experience, decided to pursue the truth by doubting everything he had so far been taught.

Milner similarly decided to set aside what she had been taught. She decided to trust not to reason but to her senses, noting, as she did so, how we defend against the passivity involved because of its cultural equation with femininity. She also noted how passive surrender arouses fear of destroying or being

[7] M. Milner (1969) *The Hands of the Living God*, London: Virago, 1988, p. xxiii.

destroyed. Nevertheless she urged herself on with the precept Conrad advanced in his novel, *Nostromo*: "to the destructive element submit yourself".[8] But she discovered there were other obstacles to surrendering herself, including being distracted by the idea of something to be attended to just ahead of the immediate moment. So, adopting a method of free association similar to that adopted by Freud from the Swedenborgian mystic, Garth Wilkinson (see p. 52), she decided to write down whatever occurred to her. She found herself writing "What I want is, not when I came to die to say, 'I've been as useful as I know how' . . . I want to feel I have 'lived'".[9] She wrote down whatever made her happy, "the important moments . . . counting over the day's spoils, little pink shells and treasures from the shore".[10]

Passively submitting to whatever occurred to her, she found herself plunging, beyond "the ripples on the surface" of her mind into the past.[11] It calmed her. But it also brought petty anxieties about the present to mind as well as past preoccupations with God, for instance. Giving way to this preoccupation, she found images of cruelty and wickedness, sin and suffering, pain and foreboding emerging.

She also discovered that, through "an internal gesture of the mind",[12] she could steer her awareness into different parts of her body, or outside of herself altogether. But this brought fear of losing herself – "of being overtaken by something".[13] Previously she had been governed by wanting to please others, by wanting scientifically to know more and more facts, and by shaping her life to "preconceived purposes".[14] Now, however, submitting to and pursuing whatever happened to occur, she began comprehending her life as the gradual discovery of a purpose she had not known.

Anticipating, in a sense, Jung's account – in his 1935 Tavistock Lectures in London – of his method of "active imagination" (see p. 88), Milner described pursuing visual images that she happened to find herself imagining. She found herself doodling – the doodle graphically expressing her discovery that, as she put it, "I could only get the most out of life by giving myself up to it".[15]

---

8 J. Field (1934) *A Life of One's Own*, London: Virago, 1986, p. 21.

9 Ibid. p. 23.

10 Ibid. p. 43.

11 Ibid. p. 59.

12 Ibid. p. 69.

13 Ibid. p. 78.

14 Ibid. p. 87.

15 Ibid. pp. 89–90.

Inspired by Lao-Tse's observation, "By non-action there is nothing which can-not be effected",[16] she decided to let go. Letting go, she discovered, entailed

> Letting the sea in . . . a deliberate negation of self . . . holding back from any form of action . . . putting something of myself out into the object I looked at so that for the moment my own will was wiped out.[17]

Playing the Montessori teacher to her thought, letting it wander wherever it would, she found she could narrow or widen her attention to focus selectively on an immediate interest or more broadly on whatever occurred. Exercising wide attention, she experienced transient moments of ineffable, noetic insight. Mystical illumination. Transforming epiphany. An example was the following:

> Once when I was lying, weary and bored with myself, on a cliff looking over the Mediterranean, I had said, "I want nothing", and immediately the landscape dropped its picture-postcard garishness and shone with a gleam from the first day of creation, even the dusty weeds by the roadside. Then again, once when ill in bed, so fretting with unfulfilled purposes that I could not at all enjoy the luxury of enforced idleness, I had found myself staring vacantly at a faded cyclamen and had happened to remem-ber to say to myself, "I want nothing". Immediately I was so flooded with the crimson of the petals that I thought I had never before known what colour was.[18]

Such moments of illumination, she discovered, could be achieved through being alert to what she called "butterflies" silently fluttering into the back of her mind.[19] But she found this could be obstructed by habit-driven "blind thinking",[20] by imposing her will on others, by equating past and present, and by self-interestedly equating thoughts and things, wishing and knowing. To gain some distance from, and separation of one from the other, she pursued visual images. She discovered a picture of a dragon she had drawn when she was 15. Free associating to it she discovered her blind thinking fed by fear of being swallowed up, and by fear of surrendering to wide attention so as "to let go and let the sea in".[21] Nevertheless she pursued these images including one of being overwhelmed by a tidal wave, by what was not her.

Since her blind thinking increased when she was tense, she taught herself to relax into her body and into whatever irritated her. With this she found the pres-ent enriched by the past flooding in. She found herself putting this in religious

---

[16] J. Field (1934) *A Life of One's Own*, London: Virago, 1986, p. 96.

[17] Ibid. p. 99.

[18] Ibid. p. 107.

[19] Ibid. p. 116.

[20] Ibid. p. 127.

[21] Ibid. p. 150.

terms. She found herself urging herself "Watch and wait . . . wait patiently for the Lord . . . Thy will, not mine, O Lord".[22] Wide attention meant being continually ready to look and accept whatever images and thoughts came, alighting, like Pegasus, as she later called Winnicott, "from places I had no knowledge of".[23]

She discovered that to think and feel herself into others, as she had into the world around her, she had to feel secure. This she discovered, she said, depended on at least once facing and letting the whole universe – everything that is not oneself – flow in and engulf one. Its precondition is accepting nothingness, wanting nothing from others. Only then can one fully experience their otherness – "the necessities of their being".[24] Summarizing her findings, she reiterated the value of looking "with a wide focus, wanting nothing and prepared for anything", without succumbing to the seemingly "endless obstacles" preventing one living with one's "eyes open".[25] She emphasized what she called the "receptive attitude to life" of eastern mysticism, without fearing that, if one is not perpetually active and efficient, as so often required of men in the west, everything one "knows and clings to will cease to exist".[26]

Reviewing Milner's book, the poet W. H. Auden applauded its culmination in "mystical experience".[27] Others welcomed its account of the healing effect of experiencing the present with the whole of one's body leading to "new knowledge . . . new contentment"; its account of "states of mind of the artist, the mystic and the lover".[28] Another writer suggested that "to feel the actuality of things", as Milner recommended, "to feel the urgency of the thing . . . is love . . . giving yourself to it".[29] The poet Stephen Spender described her message as one of "rebirth" through "spiritual virginity".[30]

More experiments in mysticism

Pursuing the life of the spirit further, Milner wrote a second book about her experiments with mysticism. She described how, lying in bed after she had

---

22 Ibid. pp. 185, 186.

23 Ibid. p. 189.

24 Ibid. p. 194.

25 Ibid. p. 199.

26 Ibid. p. 213.

27 Ibid. p. 220.

28 Ibid. pp. 221, 222.

29 Ibid. p. 224.

30 S. Spender (1934) The road to happiness, *The Spectator*, 23 November, pp. 11–12, 12.

given birth to her son and letting images flow freely in her mind, she found herself repeating the name of a book of short stories, *The Runagates Club*. It reminded her of Virginia Woolf's account of one of her characters, Mrs Dalloway, plagued with loathing of a religious zealot – "It rasped her, though, to have stirring about in her this brutal monster! . . . at any moment the brute would be stirring, this hatred".[31] This reminded Milner of a drawing she had done at the zoo, of the words "Green Wildebeste", and of a story in *The Runagate's Club* about an antiquarian unearthing a ritual for invoking God and then being destroyed in a mysterious altar fire. This in turn returned Milner full circle to childbirth, labour pains, and to how, feeling frightened, she

> Plunged deliberately into a lower darker level of awareness, dimly feeling myself part of a dark swirling current, sinking down into my body, with half thoughts of dark earth and bursting seeds, the bark of trees, the strains of rising sap.[32]

She drew a map of her life experiences, and found herself impelled to include in it a pair of horns in the background. They reminded her of folk dancers carrying antlers above their heads. She asked herself why she again and again found herself dwelling on images of a horned beast or god. Pursuing these images, she found herself writing to a lover:

> After the misery of the week-end I came to see you, submerged and hoping nothing. . . I'd come empty, expecting nothing – is that why you were able to fill me? . . . this morning I thought it would have gone, but it hasn't, I'm still possessed by you, myself is only a shell, the living thing in it is you. I'm an empty shell filled with the sound of the sea, brimming with it. Is this the losing of oneself, the self-forgetfulness that so many hunt after? . . . I'm glad, glad to be possessed, possessed by something that has no consideration for my good. I feel exultant because my good has been wiped out, for I was utterly tired of striving for my own good.[33]

With this thought came the discovery that mystical surrender entailed opening herself to what might be bad as well as good, to the Devil as well as to God.

Undaunted, she continued to pursue the method of wiping herself out, akin to that quoted by William James from St Paul, "only when I become as nothing can God enter in" (see p. 27). Telling herself, "I am nothing, I know nothing, I want nothing",[34] she found anxiety giving way to serenity, happiness, and to new and useful thinking about problems with which she had been struggling. She cited favourably other books about mysticism, as well as Freud's preface to

---

[31] Field 1937 p. 23.

[32] Ibid. p. 24.

[33] Ibid. pp. 31, 32.

[34] Ibid. p. 40.

Groddeck's *The Book of the IT* noting how the ego can be " 'lived' by unknown and uncontrollable forces".[35]

She asked herself about the force driving her to fall in love with men who "could be both fierce and gentle" and to live "parasitically" in and through them, rather than acknowledge these traits in herself.[36] She asked herself how she could trust to the self in her that could be fierce as well as gentle, and to the self that was not all "clear-headed" reason and purpose.[37] She went to a bull-fight and found herself asking herself how to give up wanting to be "the matador, in perfect mastery of the situation, wielding the sword".[38] How could she find in herself the faithful beloved, Solveig, of Ibsen's play, *Peer Gynt*, "the mother of thoughts, of true imagination"?[39] – only, she discovered, by "repeated giving up of every kind of purpose, plunging into the void".[40] Only then, she argued, "can the human spirit grow".[41]

With this she found herself approvingly quoting Blake: "What is the joy of heaven but improvement in the things of the spirit?".[42] It meant refusing to go along with those who, following Freud, rejected religion as retreat to infantile "pleasure principle" functioning.[43] It meant pursuing what might be useful in religion as means of symbolizing, dramatizing, and thereby discovering more about inner reality. Otherwise one risks remaining inhibited from discovering the truth – inside or out – for fear of being overwhelmed by infantile feelings lacking symbolic shape or form.

Going beyond the "usual vague chatter", brooding over "the memory of an experience . . . in a curious expectant stillness", she found herself, she said, "deeply rooted in the whole of my body, whereas the casual images that flitted in and out . . . seemed to belong to the head only".[44] She called the deeply rooted images "organic". Unlike conscious reasoning they "brought meaning and order into the chaos of raw feeling".[45] Organic images included making

----

[35] Ibid. p. 58.

[36] Ibid. p. 91.

[37] Ibid. p. 94.

[38] Ibid. p. 121.

[39] Ibid. p. 130.

[40] Ibid. p. 135.

[41] Ibid. p. 135.

[42] Ibid. p. 137.

[43] Ibid. p. 137.

[44] Ibid. p. 153.

[45] Ibid. p. 159.

love which, she speculated, for women at least, is often "the nearest analogy to mystical experience".[46] Or, she said, citing examples from William James, evidently "symbols of mysticism could be used as a substitute for sex".[47] Motherhood too can serve as an organic image of surrender to the "not-self"[48] – which, in turn, can figure variously as a "beast" or "god".[49] Through drawing whatever occurred to her, she discovered, she said, that the force by which one is lived can be trusted.

Just as Simone Weil likened oneness with another to parallel lines meeting at infinity (see p. 101), Milner described surrendering to what is beyond oneself in terms of the vanishing point in geometry. Surrendering to it, she found, one becomes less dependent on the actual presence of those one loves. One becomes more able to let them have lives of their own. Perhaps, she speculated, this is harder for women. She quoted Otto Weininger (the man whose writings about bisexuality were the cause of the final break between Freud and Fliess). She quoted Weininger saying, "Woman is always living in a condition of fusion with everything she knows".[50]

But whereas Weininger was an out-and-out mysogynist, Marion Milner was much more friendly to her sex. Women's experience of being inhabited by someone other than themselves in being pregnant, she said, makes them more attuned to mysticism, to surrendering to a "god-like" other.[51] But she also noted that, like men, women too may resist such self-surrender for fear of being at "the mercy of past and future . . . memories and forebodings".[52] Or they may feel swept into a "sense of nothingness, into finding their whole life in something outside themselves".[53] But therein, warned Milner, lies the danger of submission to "the reach-me-down mass-produced mythology of Hollywood, of the newspaper, or the propaganda of dictators"; better to find one's own daemon, God, or "pantheon of vital images, a mythology of one's own".[54]

---

46 Field 1937 p. 168.

47 Ibid. p. 169.

48 Ibid. p. 177.

49 Ibid. p. 179.

50 Ibid. p. 210.

51 Ibid. p. 212.

52 Ibid. p. 194–5.

53 Ibid. p. 213.

54 Ibid. p. 233.

Schoolgirl experiments

Having described the risks to women of not surrendering to mystical experience, Milner turned in her next book to findings from NIIP research she had begun in 1933 into the spiritual well-being of schoolgirls. She noted the resistance of several of the 15-year-olds she interviewed to oneness with their inner world, to what some, she said, call "submission to the Will of God and the Inner Light".[55]

She illustrated the schoolgirls' varying acceptance of, and resistance to mystical inner–outer fusion in terms of their free associations to a number of picture postcards she showed them. One was a reproduction of Frederick Walker's 1872 painting, *The Harbour of Refuge*. Another was a reproduction of John Pettie's 1884 painting, *The Vigil*. One girl, Letitia, said of the first picture, "[I] shouldn't like to be a nun – you can't do anything". She reacted to the second picture by saying, "it's pointless, I don't see what there is in it".[56] Another girl, Nesta, said the first picture was "too boring", and the second was a "silly idea altogether".[57] Still another girl, Liz, liked the first picture because it was sad, and the second because it involved "kneeling down in a lovely big place".[58] Another girl, Ann, also liked *The Vigil* because, she said, it was "so solemn and alone".[59]

Milner also asked the girls to attend to, and write down their daydreams. Some were outward-looking. Letitia wrote, "I imagine I am diving in the Olympic Games, and doing extraordinary fancy dives absolutely perfectly".[60] Others were more inward-looking. 14-year-old Laura, who liked both pictures – the "scenery" of the first, and the second because it was "peaceful and still"[61] – imagined:

> I am far away in some unknown land. . . . The fountains play and in their spray there forms a cottage smallest of the small . . . This place, once a home, is now an empty shell. The roses pink and white have spread over the doorway so that I cannot enter in. I know what is inside because through the lattice windows lovely visions play across my mind. The house is mine. . . . I call it the Home of the Unknown.[62]

---

55 M. Milner (1938) *The Human Problem in Schools*, London: Methuen, p. 162.

56 Ibid. p. 99.

57 Ibid. p. 131.

58 Ibid. p. 124.

59 Ibid. p. 137.

60 Ibid. p. 109.

61 Ibid. p. 100.

62 Ibid. pp. 109–10.

Milner concluded from the difficulties of these and other girls she interviewed that their well-being depended on combining inward-looking acceptance of what is empty and unknown with outward-looking striving. But this is only possible, she said, provided their independence and free will are recognized and valued rather than coerced. Otherwise all they can do is resist as happened, she said, to a 16-year-old, Adelaide, criticized by her teachers for not answering questions to which she knew the answers. Adelaide explained that she did this because at least it gave her the satisfaction of doing something if only by doing nothing.

Child analysis

Milner's book about her schoolgirl findings was published in 1938. The same year she met the paediatrician and psychoanalyst, Donald Winnicott, through attending one of his public lectures. She persuaded him to take on her husband, Dennis, despite his asthma, for analysis. She too went into analysis – with Sylvia Payne – and, to avoid having to become a "Cooper's Snooper", a psychologist in Duff Cooper's War Ministry, she applied and was accepted for psychoanalytic training beginning in 1940. Her supervisors included Melanie Klein. She also observed Winnicott's Saturday morning clinics for mothers and babies, and became close friends with him.

She had reservations, however, about psychoanalysis more generally. Adopting Samuel Butler's observation, "a misgiving is a warning from God to be attended to as a man values his soul",[63] she kept a diary of her misgivings. She also found herself inspired by Blake's illustrations to the *Book of Job*, depicting Job's loss of his creativity through dividing his inner and outer worlds, and becoming healed through uniting them. She drew on this image in thinking about her first psychoanalytic patient, a 17-year-old who, having been an infant prodigy at the violin, had lost his creativity in becoming almost entirely paralyzed from playing.

She called the transforming effect of uniting inner and outer reality "cosmic bliss".[64] She described how interpreting the difficulties of an 11-year-old patient, Simon, and his battles with her about the timing of his sessions, in Kleinian terms of her being an attacked and bullied inner version of his mother did little to help. His analysis only progressed, she found, when, as he began to

[63] M. Milner (1987) *The Suppressed Madness of Sane Men*, London: Tavistock, p. 9.

[64] M. Milner (1952) Aspects of symbolism in comprehension of the not-self, *IJPA*, **34** pp. 181–95, in Milner 1987 p. 95.

improve following his form-master agreeing to his holding meetings of his photography club in school, she realized that his difficulties at school might have been due to his previously experiencing it as too separate from him. Its "unmitigated not-me-ness",[65] she said, compounded the separateness he had suffered on losing his favourite woolly rabbit toy, and on his father going away to the war just when Simon's younger brother was born.

Understanding Simon's upset in Kleinian terms of his imagining and treating Milner as though she were his lost rabbit did not feel right. It implied that he experienced a clear and separate boundary between himself and others when, in fact, he often seemed to want to experience them as one. As evidence Milner described a ritual he repeatedly conducted by candlelight in his sessions with her. Blurring all boundaries between them, she said, he set her imagination alight by heating dried leaves he chose from special plants in her garden together with other ingredients in a metal cup over an electric fire. Stirring the mixture continuously, he would sometimes add a lead soldier to be melted down as a sacrifice. It became a symbol, she wrote, of his becoming reanimated through melting down and, as it were, bringing together as one his inner and outer world experience of himself and others.

Writing more generally, she cited the art critic, Berenson, describing creativity in the visual arts as involving us, its spectators, feeling one with the works of art we look at. She also noted Wordsworth's account of infancy as a time when we experience everything outward in nature as though it were within us. Perhaps, she concluded, creativity and psychological aliveness generally involve recovering an infantile illusion of inner–outer oneness with our mothers and outer reality.

Simon's problems, she argued, arose from this experience not occurring sufficiently often, or not at the right time, when he was a baby. His mother had insufficient milk. Furthermore, because the nurse often did not prepare his supplementary bottle in time, there was often a distressing gap between the beginning and end of his feed. This could have resulted in the "cosmic bliss" of being one with his mother – in wanting milk, and her providing it – turning into "catastrophic chaos". Simon, however, defended against the chaos threatened by deprivation of the illusion of inner–outer oneness with his mother by becoming prematurely separate from her, and from others. To become well, Milner accordingly argued, he had to recover this illusion.

As evidence she cited his fire cup game. She also cited his saying, towards the end of his analysis, that, when he grew up and earned his own living, he would

---

[65] Ibid. p. 93.

buy her a papier mâché clock. It would be papier mâché, he said, because she had an ornament – a little Indian dog – made of it. He had also tried unsuccessfully to make papier mâché bowls with her. Papier mâché, as Milner understood it, represented his feeling that what he found most helpful in his analysis with her was her making it into a setting in which it was safe illusorily to fuse with, mould, and treat her as though she were one with him so he could bear to recognize her and external reality generally – including the reality of time – as separate from and other than himself. With this he no longer felt so driven to try to bully others into conforming with his will, as he had in his initial battles with her over the timing of his sessions with her.

Experiments with art

Simon making papier mâché bowls in his analysis returns me to Milner's own creativity. Her mother enjoyed painting and drawing. So did her mother's father, Charles Maynard. He was a Royal Academician artist. Marion's own art – her nature sketches in her pre-teen and teenage diaries – was a form of therapy, an outward-looking means of allaying her anxiety about her father's inward-looking breakdown into schizophrenia. As a young woman, as well as doing scientific research and vocational guidance for NIIP, she attended Bernard Meninsky's evening classes in Westminster Art School.[66]

Inspired by an exhibition of free association paintings by the psychoanalyst, Grace Palethorpe, she did doodles in her analysis with Sylvia Payne. When her son was 17, she began attending residential Easter and Summer painting schools where she was taught by Cedric Morris (who also taught Lucian Freud). She continued to attend these events for the next ten years, despite deploring Morris's extreme realism and insistence that she should not paint from imagination. She much preferred the approach of another teacher, Marian Bohusz, whose classes at the Polish art school in London she attended with Winnicott's analysand and later colleague, Masud Khan.[67] Bohusz's approach was less literal than that of Morris. It informed the work she put together for a 1971 West End exhibition of her art.

Bohusz encouraged his students to play, as she had long done in her diary-keeping experiments with mysticism. She included some of the results in her fourth book, *On Not Being Able to Paint*. She began it, she said, the day war was declared. To avoid having to wear gas masks, which would have been bad

---

66 Other students included the children's book illustrator, Edward Ardizzone.

67 M. Khan (1988) Genius is energy, *Winnicott Studies*, no. 3, pp. 55–6.

for Dennis with his asthma (from which, after separating from Marion, he eventually died in 1954), they had moved to Sussex. Just as, in her previous books, she had recounted the results of letting one's thoughts wander freely, she described doing the same with drawing and painting. Depicting the Sussex Downs, she found a blazing heath emerged, quite opposite to "the moods and ideas intended".[68] Drawing chairs, she found she wanted to express feelings coming from the sense of touch and muscular movement rather than from the separation and distance of seeing. It made her think of being together with someone else, yet also separate, with different "memories and hopes and ideas".[69] It made her think of the object-otherness of the things one draws, of their existing in their own right, independent of any usefulness they might serve. Drawing things together – two jugs, for instance, side by side – the lines between them indistinct, lost in shadow, reminded her of fear of letting go to being one with another, of losing oneself in them, and of rigidly defending against any such loss of oneself through drawing firm lines as it were between oneself and them.

She described painting as "a plunge [into the outer world] that one could sometimes do deliberately but which also sometimes just happened, as when one falls in love".[70] The origin of this oneness, she said, resides in infancy when "the breast that satisfies us and the hunger that it satisfies are a mystical unity".[71] She quoted Plato on imagining one's beloved as "divine". But, she went on,

> though it is an illusion when one thinks one has found the exact embodiment of that goodness ["of what we love most"] in the external world, since outer reality is never permanently the same as our dreams, yet such moments are the vital illusion by which we live.[72]

Such moments are transforming. They change our dreams through making us want and act to bring the "transfigured" person or thing nearer to us.[73]

But this raises the problem that dreams can involve monsters as well as gods. Once one endows external objects with the "spiritual life" of one's dreams they can become infernal. Or one might stop others having their own "spiritual identity" for lack of being able to be oneself.[74] Fearful of losing faith in the

---

[68] M. Milner (1950) *On Not Being Able to Paint*, Madison, CT: International Universities Press, 1957, p. 8.

[69] Ibid. p. 14.

[70] Ibid. p. 26.

[71] Ibid. p. 27.

[72] Ibid. p. 29.

[73] Ibid. p. 30.

[74] Ibid. p. 43.

existence of goodness, one may defend against disappointment of the illusion of oneness of subject and object. One may defend against fear of separation, and fear of losing those one loves, by seeking to envelop and merge with them. But this risks destroying them, or us. Hence fear of the mystical union involved in "plunging into experiences where the boundaries of personal identity are transcended".[75]

Nevertheless Milner found her most expressive drawings came from just such quasi-mystical "dreamy states of mind".[76] Experimenting with free drawing, she found "dreams and reality" coming together again.[77] Their coming together involves hatred as well as love – hatred of the external world for not living up to one's dreams and expectations. Achieving a work of art, she went on, depends on a "state of grace" enabling the artist to exalt and describe the world around him.[78] It involves both body and spirit, oneness in "twoness", realized imagination, "like the sun coming out over a world that had been all greyness".[79]

If one loses hope of any such illuminating oneness with others we may deny needing them, retreat into unexpressed dreams, or let ourselves be dictated to and conform with their demands. By contrast, through free drawing, Milner found herself engaging with outer reality as pliant and undemanding. Endowing people and things with spiritual life, she discovered through painting and drawing, entailed selecting those details that emphasize the "soul".[80] She thereby found herself gaining a firmer hold on the spiritual reality of her gods, on what she loved and wanted to cherish, and on what she hated and wanted to expunge. And she discovered this thinking in pictures was instantaneous. It brought the past into a single, present, solid moment. Through painting and drawing she discovered, she said, that:

> The experience of outer and inner coinciding, which we blindly undergo when we fall in love, is consciously brought about in the arts, through the conscious acceptance of the as-if-ness of the experience and the conscious manipulation of a malleable material.[81]

Art neither denies inner dreams nor outer reality, including the conventions of its time and place.

---

75 M. Milner (1950) *On Not Being Able to Paint*, Madison, CT: International Universities Press, p. 66.

76 Ibid. p. 71.

77 Ibid. p. 86.

78 Ibid. p. 106

79 Ibid. pp. 111, 112.

80 Ibid. p. 120.

81 Ibid. p. 131.

Bringing together the twoness of inner and outer, subject and object, depends, Milner discovered, on what she called "contemplative action".[82] It depends, she argued, on the "willingness in our original environment of persons, in the actual home of our infancy, to fit in with our dreams".[83] It depends on not being catastrophically disillusioned in discovering that what we make, in the first place shit, is not as lovely as the feelings we put into giving it to others. Treatment of the resulting inhibitions accordingly entails, said Milner, battling over "the 'language' of love . . . over the way in which the orgasm, or the orgastic experiences, are to be symbolised" without being repudiated.[84] The precondition of creativity and mental health and life, she concluded, contrary to Freud, is the "oceanic feeling . . . 'emptiness' as a beneficent state . . . [as] in the *Tao Te Ching* . . . the satisfied sleep of the infant at the mother's breast . . . ecstasy and elation".[85] Art gives new form to feeling. It involves, she said, what Stokes called "out-there-ness".[86] Its precondition, she concluded, is "a setting in which it is safe to indulge in reveries, safe to permit a con-fusion of 'me' and 'not-me' ".[87]

Art therapy

Milner arguably learnt much of this not only from using painting and drawing in her own self-analysis but also from using art therapy in her psychoanalysis of a schizophrenic patient, Susan. Winnicott's wife, Alice, had been struck by Susan's beauty in the hospital where Susan was a patient. She looked, said Alice, "like the Botticelli Venus rising from the waves".[88] Appalled by her subsequent "terrible state" after having electro-convulsive therapy (ECT), Alice persuaded Susan to come and live with her and Winnicott and he referred her for treatment with Milner.

Her treatment began on 17 November 1943. She was then 23. She arrived, "tall and slim", wrote Milner, "with a walk like Garbo in *Queen Christina* and a remotely withdrawn madonna-like face".[89] She told Milner she had lost her

---

[82] Ibid. p. 140.

[83] Ibid. p. 138.

[84] Ibid. p. 151.

[85] Ibid. p. 154.

[86] Ibid. p. 160.

[87] Ibid. p. 165.

[88] Milner 1969 p. 3.

[89] Ibid. p. 3.

soul, that the world was no longer outside her, and that this had all happened since she had had ECT three weeks before. It had made her lose all sense of reality, and all sense of herself in the world. Before that she had been doing war work for four years on a farm to which she had persuaded a friend, Jackie, to take her. She had met Jackie in a dance troupe, in which she worked after doing a number of other jobs, after drifting away from school when she was 14.

Shortly before her breakdown Susan had fallen in love with a young sculptor who was also doing war work on the farm. She had also suffered the shock of discovering Jackie's mother, Mrs Dick – a semi-invalid whom everyone loathed and whom Susan alone had looked after – dead in bed from a heart attack. Susan reacted by suffering acute pains in her heart, and by being constantly sick. In thus seemingly imagining herself to be one with Mrs Dick, she also felt, as she put it, that she was one with the world. She called it "breaking down into reality".[90]

For the first time in her life, she felt she was "in the world": she discovered that she was in her body, that space existed, that if she walked away from things they got farther away; and she discovered that she had not made herself . . . her emotions were "absolutely terrific" because she was getting into the world for the first time.[91]

During this period of her life, she later said, she was a "mystic".[92] The experience taught her, said Milner, the meaning of St Paul's reference to "the length and breadth and depth and height of the love of God".[93] But she could no longer work on the farm. Her friend, Jackie, lost interest in her, and sent her away to live with someone else, from where, six weeks later, she was admitted to mental hospital.

Reconstructing Susan's story in analysis, it transpired that her mother had been mad. She had brought up Susan and her older sister single-handed. Susan only learnt later that the lodger, Jack, was her father. He first came to live with them after being invalided out of the army when Susan was learning to walk. Later, when she was 4, an old man living next door began bribing her with bread and jam and sweets to let him masturbate against her. When she eventually told her mother, her mother protested, "Don't tell me – it will kill me!" So Susan said no more.

Her mother idealized her. She called her "O moon of my delight". She told her, "I love you the whole world".[94] She had Susan sleep in the same bed with

[90] Milner 1969 p. 9.

[91] Ibid. p. 9.

[92] Milner 1989 p. 259.

[93] Ibid. p. 264.

[94] Milner 1969 p. 5.

her till Susan was 14. She could not bear for Susan to be separate or different from her. She insisted they were the same. After Susan had ECT she crowed: "Now you are mad and so am I!"[95] But she also blamed all the family's troubles on Susan, from which Susan concluded that her mother wished she had never been born.

Faced with the dangerousness of reviving the infantile illusion of being one with her mother, given that her mother seemingly wished her dead, Susan's analysis entailed making it safe for her to revive this illusion of oneness with another. This entailed enabling Susan to experience oneness with Milner, without going mad as she had in her mystical experience of being one with the world around her when she fell in love and when she identified with the chest pains of the dead Mrs Dick. But Susan rigidly defended against experiencing any such oneness with Milner in so far as she experienced her, as she had her mother, as annihilating or mad.

Nor could she abide becoming alive to, and one with the unconscious forces by which she was lived. She rejected the notion of unconscious symbolism: "A thing is what it is and can't be anything else", she insisted.[96] She could not bear to be aware of inner reality, so much had she had to keep an eye on outer reality when she was an infant for fear of what her mother might do to her. Her tragedy, as Milner saw it, was to have both experienced and lost her mother as a reliable and all-enveloping god. Milner accordingly called her book about Susan's treatment after one of D. H. Lawrence's Pascalian *pensées* or pansy poems: "It is a fearful thing to fall into the hands of the living God. / But it is a much more fearful thing to fall out of them".[97]

Perhaps, Milner thought, it was something of the mystical experience of her mother's hands and arms holding, sustaining, and protecting her, God-like, without which she would have died as a baby, that recurred when, as Susan put it, she suddenly felt alive – at one in her body and in the world – before having ECT.

During the first years of Susan's analysis Milner also went into analysis, this time with Winnicott. So as not to muddle it up with her analysis of Susan, she was analysed by him in her home rather than in his home where Susan lived. But his analysing her in her home was not very satisfactory, and soon after her analysis began Winnicott told her it had to stop whereupon, it seems, she burst into tears. Perhaps it was her upset at her analysis with Winnicott ending that led Milner to go briefly into analysis with Clifford Scott. The same year, 1949,

---

95 Ibid. p. 14.

96 Ibid. p. 40.

97 Ibid. p. 52.

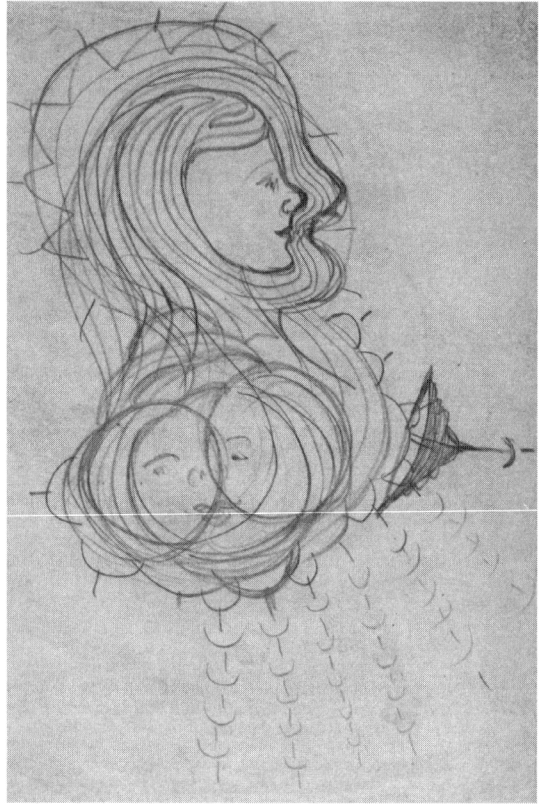

Fig. 9.1 Overlapping circles.

the Winnicotts separated. During the breakup of their marriage Susan felt too insecure to revive the infantile illusion of oneness with others involved in allowing herself, as Milner put it, "to go to pieces in order to come together in a new way".[98] But she felt more secure after going to live with an elderly woman friend of the Winnicotts, and after she began paying for her analysis – a nominal shilling a session – now that Winnicott no longer paid for it.

Perhaps it was her analysis no longer being so muddled up with the Winnicotts that freed Susan, beginning in early March 1950, to start doing doodles and drawings in her analysis with Milner. They included a picture of an angel and of a devil representing Milner; a picture of Milner as both an outside and inside, fused and separate, moon mother to her; a drawing of a placenta, which Milner interpreted as indicating her wanting Milner to

[98] Milner 1969 p. 59.

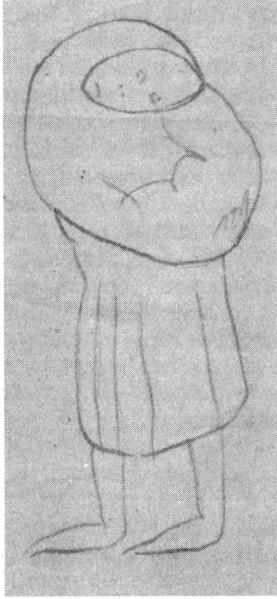

Fig. 9.2 Cradling figure.

provide her with "an eternity of unbroken fusion and continuity of existence";[99] and drawings of alternating "oneness" and "twoness", including circles which can be seen as one face or two (see Fig. 9.1).[100]

Eventually she brought a picture she had drawn years before after having ECT. In it she depicted herself as both one with, and separate from an androgynous, god-like figure cradling her (see Fig. 9.2).[101] Slowly she became aware of being cradled and held by her body. She drew ducks held and supported by water. Soon after, on 8 January 1959, she announced, "I am in the world for the first time in sixteen years".[102] If only, said Milner, she had found a hostel where she could have got help when she first experienced herself "breaking down into reality",[103] it might have not taken her so long to become psychologically alive again. Milner prefaced her 1969 book about Susan with the hope that it would contribute to improving mental health provision, so that others would not suffer as Susan had following her wartime mystical experience of being one with the world around her.

....

[99] Ibid. p. 102.

[100] Ibid. p. 163.

[101] Ibid. p. 251.

[102] Ibid. p. 375.

[103] Ibid. p. 9.

She wrote about Susan's doodles and drawings in an essay about psycho-analysis and mysticism, in which she also referred to a book by Suzuki, *Essays in Zen Buddhism*, which Simone Weil likewise enjoyed over thirty years before.[104] In particular, Milner referred to an image of a blank circle in Suzuki's book which, she said, evoked consciousness uniting mind and body by wholly suffusing the latter from within. The image of the blank circle also reminded her of her diary-keeping formula – "I have nothing, I know nothing, I want nothing" – which, she said, she had initially abandoned on training to become a psychoanalyst because she had then thought it to be a pathological defence against reality. Now, however, she again asserted that, far from being a sign of illness, embracing nothingness can be a means to health.

Final mysticism and art therapy

Milner included essays about mysticism in a book called *The Suppressed Madness of Sane Men* after a phrase coined by William James' Harvard colleague, George Santayana, in likening mysticism to madness. In her book she noted how, in staring at an object without thinking of using it, a change in one's whole body perception emerges along with a move toward interest in the sheer "thusness" – the separation and unique identity – of the thing stared at.[105] Some, she said, cannot bear the aloneness involved. Others, Susan for instance, are driven mad by, and therefore defend against, mystical inner–outer oneness with the formlessness of their being. For they feel that everything inside their being is lost and destroyed.

Milner herself, however, continued to engage in experiments with mysticism. Her findings were published in a book she called after a poem by Blake:

> He who binds to himself a joy
> Doth the winged life destroy
> But he who kisses the joy as it flies
> Lives in Eternity's sunrise.[106]

In her book she detailed incidents from her travels in Italy, Canada, Spain, Greece, France, Corsica, Ibiza, Kashmir and Israel. She told these incidents as though they were the "memory beads", as she put it, of a rosary. They included

[104] "*Je te recommande les ouvrages du philosophe Teitaro Suzuki sur le boudhism Zen, en anglais; c'est extrêmement curieux*", to Simone Pétrement, 26 February 1942, in S. Weil (1942) *Œuvres Complètes tome VI: Cahiers 8–12 [February to July 1942], La porte du transcendant*, Paris: Gallimard, 2002, p. 37.

[105] M. Milner (1977) Winnicott and overlapping circles, in Milner 1987 pp. 279–86, 282.

[106] M. Milner (1987) *Eternity's Sunrise*, London: Virago, p. vi.

an image of Giorgione's painting, *The Tempest*, depicting, said Milner, a woman's awareness bound neither to a man nor to her child. Another image was of recovering the monumental and eternal wisdom of the goddess of the Parthenon through thinking herself into the heaviness of its stone women – the Caryatids. She recalled fear of all support failing, and recovering through dwelling on the protective enveloping cloak of Piero della Francesca's *Our Lady of Mercy*. In an interview launching the book, she also dwelt on the mystical inner–outer oneness evoked by memory of herself as a child at school singing, "On the Resurrection morning soul and body meet again".[107]

Resurrection through creatively reviving oneness with others included, for Milner in old age, putting together bits and pieces from her previously discarded paintings to make new collages. One was of her and her brother. She called it *We Two Together*. It reminded her, she said, of the time when, as children, they imagined marrying each other. One of her last public engagements was to attend the installation at Imperial College of a statue of him by Epstein. Through her final years she attended seminars at London's Squiggle Foundation devoted to the work of Winnicott.

In the late 1970s she had been Honorary President of the British Association of Art Therapists. Many years later, on the evening of 28 May 1998, a member of the Association visited her. Susan and Winnicott were much on her mind. She wept and, out of her distress, found a last line for a chapter about Winnicott to be included in another book of associations to drawings, those of her son when he was a child.[108] But the book, called *Bothered by Alligators*, was not published in her lifetime. That night she died, spared the realization of her doctor's prophecy that she would live to repeat the beginning of another century. Nevertheless her work lives on in many psychoanalysts and psychotherapists, like her, seeking to enable their patients to recover the oneness with another experienced by some as divine which, according to William James, lies at the heart of what is best and most therapeutic in religion.

---

[107] A. Karpf (1987) Experiment in leisure, The *Observer*, 8 February, p. 54.

[108] M. Thompson (2000) Appreciation of Marion Milner, in L. Caldwell (ed.) *Art, Creativity, Living*, London: Karnac, pp. 144–6.

Chapter 10

Donald Winnicott

Transitional transcendence

Marion Milner emphasized the healing effects of recovering the illusion of oneness with another involved in mystical and religious experience. But where do our illusions, fantasies and dreams come from in the first place? Klein argued that they stem from inborn instincts of love and hate. Donald Winnicott, by contrast, argued that they are first given life and content by our mothers' psychological oneness with us as babies. This, he also argued, is the precondition of the baby's subsequent experience of being both one with, and separate from his mother. Winnicott described this experience as occurring in what he called a "transitional", "potential", or "third area" between subject and object, me and not-me, that he and his followers locate as the source of transcendence and religious experience, which he assimilated to playing. It is with this that I will begin.

Playing

Preoccupied with playing, Winnicott began one of his last essays quoting the Indian poet and educationalist, Rabindranath Tagore: "On the seashore of endless worlds, children play".[1] Actually Tagore said "meet" not "play".[2] But meeting was much the same for Winnicott. Like the children in Tagore's poem, he grew up near the sea. Born in Plymouth on 7 April 1896, he was the youngest of three children in a prosperous, Wesleyan Methodist family. Many years later his widow, Clare, described his childhood home – large house, spacious grounds, lots of love – as idyllic, adding: "Some . . . may be inclined to think that it sounds too good to be true. But the truth is that it *was* good".[3]

---

[1] D. W. Winnicott (1967) The location of cultural experience, in D. W. Winnicott (1971) *Playing and Reality*, Harmondsworth: Penguin, 1974, pp. 112–21, 112.

[2] R. Tagore (1912) *Gitanjali*, London: Macmillan, 1921 p. 54.

[3] In C. Winnicott (1978) D. W. W.: A reflection, in S. A. Grolnick *et al.* (eds) *Between Reality and Fantasy*, New York: Jason Aronson, pp. 17–33, 25.

Winnicott too remembered it as idyllic. He remembered, for instance, his parents so well imagining what he might want that one Christmas he woke up to discover that they had given him exactly what he wanted without his even knowing such things existed – "a blue cart made in Switzerland, like those that the people there use for bringing home wood".[4] But he also had less good memories – a memory, for instance, of himself, as a child, having to enliven his mother from depression:

> Once, stretched out on her lap
> as now on dead tree
> I learned to make her smile
> to stem her tears
> to undo her guilt
> to cure her inward death
> To enliven her was my living.[5]

He also recalled that when he was 9, as his analysand, friend, and colleague, Masud Khan put it, "suddenly he decided to louse it all up, and so messed up his copybooks and did badly in examinations for a year".[6]

Later, when Winnicott was 12, his father, annoyed at his using bad language, and blaming it on the company he was keeping, or so said Winnicott, decided to send him to boarding school. Winnicott started there when he was 13. It was a Wesleyan school, The Leys, in Cambridge. Here Winnicott first read Darwin's *The Origin of Species* – "I could not leave off reading it . . . it showed that living things could be examined scientifically with the corollary that gaps in knowledge and understanding need not scare me."[7] Breaking his collar bone playing games, he decided to become a doctor, otherwise, he said, "for the rest of my life I should have to depend on doctors if I damaged myself or became ill".[8] He went to Jesus College, Cambridge, to study the necessary biology, served as a ship's doctor during the war (reading Henry James' novels in his spare time), and afterwards completed his medical training at St Bartholomew's Hospital in London.

---

[4] D. W. Winnicott (1962) Providing for the child in health and in crisis, in D. W. Winnicott (1965) *The Maturational Processes and the Facilitating Environment*, London: Hogarth, pp. 64–72, 70.

[5] Poem by Winnicott in A. Phillips (1988) *Winnicott*, London: Fontana, p. 29.

[6] M. Khan (1975) Introduction, in D. W. Winnicott (1958) *Collected Papers*, London: Karnac, pp. xi-l, xxxvi.

[7] D. W. Winnicott (1945) Towards an objective study of human nature, in D. W. Winnicott (1996) *Thinking about Children*, Reading, Mass: Addison-Wesley, pp. 3–12, 7.

[8] In Winnicott 1978 p. 25.

Here, in London, having attended the Methodist church regularly in Cambridge, Winnicott converted to Anglicanism. Bothered by having lost the ability, after the war, to remember his dreams, he also discovered psychoanalysis through reading a book about it by Freud's Swiss pastor friend, Oskar Pfister. Writing enthusiastically about Freud's book, *The Interpretation of Dreams*, to one of his sisters, he told her how much he appreciated psychoanalysts, unlike hypnotists, seeking to enable their patients to think for themselves. At the risk of blaspheming, he said, Christ too was just such "a leading psychotherapist".[9]

In 1920 Winnicott qualified as a doctor and, having been fascinated by children during his medical training, decided to specialize in paediatrics, in which he got a job at Paddington Green Children's Hospital (where he worked for the next forty years). With money from his father, he also set up in private practice near Harley Street, and the same year married a slightly older, fellow Cambridge graduate, Alice Buxton Taylor, on 7 July 1923, with whom he settled in Surbiton.

Alice was a potter. She also suffered with mental illness, and their marriage was evidently rather unhappy. Perhaps this contributed to Winnicott going into analysis, beginning in the autumn of 1924, with James Strachey. It enabled him, he said, to have "healing dreams".[10] He also learnt from Strachey about Klein's work, and, through supervision with her, came to admire her "way of making inner psychic reality very real".[11]

More free-thinking than Klein, perhaps in part because of his non-conformist upbringing, Winnicott seemed less constricted by theory in imagining himself into the inner world of the children he treated. Examples abound. In his first book, for instance, he described a 1-year-old referred on account of seeming epileptic fits. At their first meeting, he noted how, sitting on his knee, she bit his knuckle, threw his spatulas on the floor, cried and then, having gone through this performance again another time, suddenly began enjoying playing. She began fingering her toes through her shoes and socks and, when Winnicott had them removed, she again and again proved with great satisfaction to herself, he said, "that whereas spatulas (and socks, I might have said) can be put to the mouth, thrown away, and lost, toes cannot be pulled off".[12]

---

[9] To Violet, 15 November 1919, in D. W. Winnicott (1987) *The Spontaneous Gesture*, Cambridge: Harvard University Press, p. 3.

[10] D. W. Winnicott (1947) Hate in the countertransference, in Winnicott 1958 pp. 194–203, 197.

[11] D. W. Winnicott (1962) A personal view of the Kleinian contribution, in Winnicott 1965 pp. 171–8, 174.

[12] D. W. Winnicott (1931) *Clinical Notes on Disorders of Children*, in Winnicott 1996 p. 265.

After that, it seems, through his having imagined himself into her fears, and enabled her to reassure herself about them through playing with him, she never had another fit. Winnicott urged his fellow-doctors similarly to imagine themselves into their infant patients' shoes, adding "I am aware that this is a rather funny figure of speech since babies are not born with shoes on, but I think you will understand my meaning".[13]

Meanwhile, in the early 1930s, Winnicott had moved with his wife, Alice, to Pilgrim's Lane in Hampstead, near their art historian and collector friend, Jim Ede (now known for the art gallery he founded in Kettle's Yard in Cambridge). Disappointed by Klein not taking him on for analysis (because she wanted him to analyse her son, Erich), Winnicott went into analysis with her colleague, Joan Riviere. In 1934 he qualified as a psychoanalyst, and the next year qualified as a child analyst. In his qualifying essay for membership of the BPAS, he emphasized the importance of psychoanalysts imaginatively entering their patients' inner world as regards religion. He warned against their dismissing their patients' belief in God as an illusion or fantasy. For, he argued, this could unjustifiably add to their patients' depression, the deadness of which he attributed to loss of faith in being able to love. He also wrote of the symbolizing of love defeating death in the despair of Good Friday followed by the manic excitement of Christ's Easter Day resurrection: "The Ascension," he concluded, "marks recovery from depression".[14]

Later, sympathizing with the plight of children separated from those they love, Winnicott wrote with others to the *British Medical Journal*, protesting against government plans to evacuate children away from their homes during the war.[15] Nevertheless the plans went ahead, and the next year Winnicott began work as a psychiatric consultant to a number of evacuation hostels established in Oxfordshire for children who could not cope with evacuation to ordinary foster families.

Lovers, children, and babies

Through his work in the hostels, which Winnicott visited on Fridays, he met and fell in love with a social worker, Clare Britton, who also worked in the

---

[13] D. W. Winnicott (1967) The bearing of emotional development on feeding problems, ibid. pp. 44–6, 45.

[14] D. W. Winnicott (1935) The manic defence, in Winnicott 1958 pp. 129–44, 135.

[15] From Bowlby, Miller and Winnicott, 16 December 1939, in D. W. Winnicott (1984) *Deprivation and Delinquency*, London: Routledge, pp. 13–14.

hostels. Soon, a friend later said, Friday became "a red-letter day" for Clare.[16] Working with him, said Clare, "was to be in a situation of complete reciprocity where giving and taking were indistinguishable".[17] She was living in a flat in Oxford where it is possible Winnicott also stayed. Certainly Clare later recalled from this time his secretly buying a whole pushcart of peonies early one morning for her to discover when she got up.[18]

In 1944 they reported their evacuation hostel findings together.[19] They described the upset of children coming into their care: their bed wetting and soiling; their ganging together in stealing; burning down haystacks; wrecking trains; running away; and sexual promiscuity. They described how, on first arriving at the hostels, the children saw the staff and other residents in terms of their inner lives and illusions about how they imagined and wanted them to be. They recounted how this was succeeded by the children testing whether those around them could physically and emotionally withstand their destructiveness. Only then, it seems, could they begin to settle down to what was actually there.[20]

Arguably inspired by love of Clare, and by his findings with her regarding the loss of psychological animation in children lacking maternal love or care,[21] Winnicott now began developing his pioneering account of the oneness of mothers with their babies as a precondition of their fantasies and illusions coming to life. In an essay first published in 1945, he emphasized that our mothers first bring us psychologically alive through loving and imagining themselves into what we might think and feel. It is this oneness, or loving identification, with her baby that enables the mother to meet and feed his dreams with details of external reality.

Drawing also on his wartime psychoanalytic work with patients suffering with psychosis, Winnicott described in this essay a stage before the baby is aware of having an inside or that his mother has an inside and can feel concerned about her. Before all this, he speculated, the baby's inner life is utterly unintegrated. Klein argued that the baby's fragmented and divided self comes

---

[16] J. Kanter (2000) The untold story of Clare and Dontald Winnicott: How social work influenced modern psychoanalysis, *Clinical Social Work Journal*, **28**(3) pp. 245–61, 250.

[17] C. Winnicott (1983) Introduction, in Winnicott 1984 pp. 1–5, 4.

[18] J. Kanter (2004) *Face-to-Face with Clare Winnicott: Her Life and Legacy*, London: Karnac.

[19] D. W. Winnicott & C. Britton (1944) The problem of homeless children, *New Era*, Sept–Oct, pp. 155–61.

[20] D. W. Winnicott and C. Britton (1947) Residential management as treatment for difficult children, in Winnicott 1984 pp. 54–72.

[21] My thanks to Joel Kanter for pointing out this aspect of Clare's influence on Winnicott.

together as an effect of an instinct of love within him. By contrast, Winnicott argued that integration comes about in the baby both through his instinctual experiences gathering him together and through his mother's oneness with him enabling her to bring him together through her emotional and physical care of him in keeping him warm, handling, bathing, rocking and naming him. As a result the baby can then begin to bear long stretches of time not minding whether he is whole or in bits.

Through her oneness with her baby enabling her to anticipate his illusions, she gives them outward reality. She feeds his illusion of having created outer reality, including his illusion of himself and her as one:

> The infant comes to the breast when excited, and ready to hallucinate something fit to be attacked. At that moment the actual nipple appears and he is able to feel it was that nipple that he hallucinated. So his ideas are enriched by actual details of sight, feel, smell, and next time this material is used in the hallucination. In this way he starts to build up a capacity to conjure up what is actually available.[22]

Indeed, said Winnicott, "it is a mother's job . . . to go on steadily providing the simplified bit of the world which the infant, through her, comes to know".[23] It involves, Winnicott added, a shared reality, constituted by "the infant's hallucinating and the world's presenting, with moments of illusion for the infant in which the two are taken by him to be identical".[24]

All this takes work. It entails the presence of someone "taking the trouble all the time to bring the world to the baby in understandable form".[25] In doing so, the mother brings about the birth of the baby's psyche or spirit. Through feeding her child's illusions, the mother brings into being his "interest in bubbles and clouds and rainbows and all mysterious phenomena", which, said Winnicott, is the basis of our "interest in breath . . . which provides a basis for the conception of spirit, soul, anima".[26]

Winnicott very much relied on Clare to inspire his ideas about these matters. Or so he said. Writing to her about a paper he was working on, he noted:

> My work is really quite a lot associated with you. Your effect on me is to make me keen and productive and this is all the more awful – because when I am cut off from you I feel paralyzed for all action and originality.[27]

....

[22] D. W. Winnicott (1945) Primitive emotional development, in Winnicott 1958 pp. 145–56, 153.

[23] Ibid. p. 153.

[24] Ibid. p. 154.

[25] Ibid. p. 154.

[26] Ibid. p. 154.

[27] To Clare, December 1946, in Winnicott 1978 p. 32.

The outcome was startlingly original. In his resulting paper, and going against the frequent sentimentalizing of therapy and mothering, he drew attention to the many reasons psychoanalysts, therapists, and mothers have for hating their patients and babies. He too could hate. He hated, he said, the 9-year-old runaway from one of the wartime evacuation hostels his wife, Alice, had invited to live with them during the war. Parents and others looking after babies and children hate them in large part, he indicated, because of all the detailed study and care involved in bringing external reality into accord with, and thus feeding and bringing alive their inner reality with details of the world around them. Analysts and mothers must know about the hatred evoked in them by their charges. Otherwise, said Winnicott, their patients and children cannot know about their own hatred of them.[28]

He described this in a talk he gave on 5 February 1947. The next year, having been bereaved of his mother in 1925, he was bereaved of his father, who died on 31 December 1948. His death, it seems, freed Winnicott to tell Alice about his relationship with Clare, and to ask her for a divorce. By early 1949, finding it too painful to return home to Alice, he often slept overnight in his consulting room. The stress however took its toll – he suffered a heart attack and had to take three months convalescent leave from his children's hospital work.

But he went on writing about our transformation into aliveness by the oneness of our mothers with us as babies. He wrote about how this oneness helps mothers protect us from our nascent "continuity of being" becoming fragmented by having to react to, or defend ourselves from inner or outer "impingement". Without such protection, he said, babies risk developing on a lifeless, compliant, "false self" basis in which the psyche simply functions to register and catalogue the impingements to which it has to react.[29]

He described the implications of this for psychoanalysis. Just as the baby's imaginative life comes into being through his mother's oneness with him enabling her to anticipate and meet what he imagines to be there through her emotional and physical care, so too the analyst may have to do this for patients deadened in their spirit and imagination by psychosis. One of his patients, Margaret Little, who first went into analysis with him in 1949, later recounted something of this understanding oneness by him occurring in her first session with him:

> I lay curled up tight, completely hidden under the blanket, unable to move or speak. D.W. was silent until the end of the hour, when he said only, "I don't know, but I have

---

[28] D. W. Winnicott (1947) Hate in the countertransference, in Winnicott 1958 pp. 194–203.

[29] D. W. Winnicott (1949) Mind and its relation to the psyche-soma, ibid. pp. 243–54.

the feeling that you are shutting me out for some reason." This brought relief, for he could admit not knowing, and could allow contradiction if it came. Much later I realized that I had been shutting myself in, taking up the smallest possible amount of space and being as unobtrusive as I could.[30]

Another time, she writes, she was seized with "recurring spasms of terror . . . grabbed his hands and clung tightly till the spasms passed".[31] Soon she discovered she spent the first half of every session taking in the silence and stillness Winnicott gave her, and extended for her by giving her almost twice the usual time for each of her sessions. Sometimes, when she was too depressed to go out, he came to see her at home. If necessary he would physically hold and bear with her distress as she wept. One time he gave her a handkerchief to comfort her over a holiday break. His "environmental provision", as he might have called it, enabled her to become alive from her previous moribund, false self, "cheap second-hand copy" of her mother.[32] She became full of the verve and life with which Winnicott enlivened their later analytic sessions together with jokes, stories, and nonsense. She became an artist and, like him, a successful analyst.

Soon after Margaret Little's analysis with Winnicott began, he gave a talk in which, perhaps thanks to his love of Clare (who, Masud Khan complained, boasted "she made Winnicott potent"),[33] he spoke publicly about sex. He described it as involving both eroticism and aggression, fusion and separation. He described both as stemming from the baby's early relation with the mother. In his excitedly aggressive love for her, he said, the baby comes up against her as someone separate outside his control. Winnicott contrasted this discovery of the separateness of others, through our own lively and aggressive love for them, with passive and lifeless responding to impingement in which the psyche can only survive, and then only in an inanimate and restricted way, through withdrawing. Or the psyche may only be able to retain a life through walling itself off from an outer self façade in an inner "true self", the existence of which depends on "not being found".[34] By contrast, Winnicott said, lovers

[30] M. Little (1990) *Psychotic Anxieties and Containment*, Northvale, NJ: Jason Aronson, pp. 42–3.

[31] Ibid. p. 43.

[32] Ibid. p. 34.

[33] In L.B. Hopkins (1998) D. W. Winnicott's analysis of Masud Khan, *Contemporary Psychoanalysis*, **34**(1) pp. 5–47, 32.

[34] D. W. Winnicott (1950) Aggression in relation to emotional development, ibid. pp. 204–18, 218.

ideally find in making love the inspiration and life of oneness or fusion and separateness in each other's "actual presence, satisfaction, and survival".[35]

Some months later – in August 1950 – Winnicott talked with Clare's brother about his involvement with Clare, and about his difficulty in getting a divorce lest it threaten her reputation as director of the child care course at the London School of Economics which she now ran. Soon after he suffered another heart attack. Previously he had written to Clare about a dream which, he said, reminded him of a doll he had as a child:

> If I love you as I loved this (must I say?) doll, I love you all out. And I believe I do. Of course I love you all sorts of other ways, but this thing came new to me. I felt enriched, and felt more like going on writing my paper on transition objects (postponed to October).[36]

Perhaps because of his heart attack the paper had to be postponed again. He did not present it till 30 May 1951.

Called "Transitional objects and transitional phenomena", the resulting essay remains, today, one of Winnicott's most important papers, not least because it concerns the transforming area of oneness in twoness central to religious experience. In his essay Winnicott wrote about an area intermediate between inner and outer reality to which, he said, both contribute. This "third area", he said, begins in infancy when the baby, in sucking his thumb, for instance, caresses his face with his fingers and, with the other hand, takes part of a sheet or blanket into his mouth, or plucks and collects wool to add to his caressing activity, all of which he may later accompany with "mum-mum" sounds, babbling, and singing. Winnicott called these activities "transitional phenomena". From them, he said, may develop a "transitional object", something soft – a blanket say – which the baby finds, and in a sense creates. It is suffused both with subjective oneness with his mother, but at the same time it is out there, objective. Winnicott called it "the first possession". It belongs, he said, to an "intermediate area between the subjective and what is objectively perceived".[37]

The baby may give this "Not-Me" object a name. Incorporating words made by grownups around him, he may call it "baa" from the "b" of "baby" or "bear".[38] He may cuddle, and excitedly love and attack it. Then it gradually loses its

---

[35] D. W. Winnicott (1950) Aggression in relation to emotional development, *Psychoanalysis*, 34(1) p. 218.

[36] To Clare, early 1950, in Winnicott 1978 p. 31.

[37] D. W. Winnicott (1951) Transitional objects and transitional phenomena, in Winnicott 1958 pp. 229–42, 231.

[38] Ibid. p. 232.

meaning. Or, rather, said Winnicott, its meaning suffuses the whole interven-ing area between the child's inner personal life and outer reality. It spreads and widens out into play, art, and religious feeling.

Religion and therapy

Winnicott stressed the variation between toddlers in their experience and use of transitional phenomena. He similarly emphasized variations between reli-gions in their symbolic elaboration of these phenomena. Illustrating the point, he wrote:

> If we consider the wafer of the Blessed Sacrament, which is symbolic of the body of Christ, I think I am right in saying that for the Roman Catholic community it *is* the body, and for the Protestant community it is a *substitute*, a reminder, and is essentially not, in fact, actually the body itself. Yet in both cases it is a symbol.[39]

To this the Catholic psychoanalyst, William Meissner,[40] adds that our religious beliefs reflect ongoing changes in this potential or transitional space in which subject and object are one. It both grounds and enriches subjectivity with the objective, material world, to which subjectivity gives transcendence. Their two-in-oneness is transforming. The material objectivity of the communion wafer grounds and enriches the subjective psyche. But the wafer would have no holiness were it not for the believer infusing and suffusing it with the life and faith of his inner psyche.

As for Winnicott, at the end of the year, 1951, in which he first presented his theory of transitional phenomena, his divorce from Alice was finalized. A couple of weeks later, on 28 December 1951, he and Clare married. She had been liv-ing in Chelsea. Now they moved to Chester Square in Belgravia. They were evidently very much in love. The psychoanalyst, Pearl King, said they "sparked each other off". The Tavistock Clinic's director, Jock Sutherland, said Clare "had a great natural empathy which filled in with (Donald's) and they did a great deal for each other". Marion Milner noted that Clare's "gifts of liveliness, sense of fun, even mischieviousness, combined with a deep seriousness, met the same in Donald Winnicott and she undoubtedly had a great influence on his work".[41]

---

[39] Ibid. p. 234.

[40] W. Meissner (1984) *Psychoanalysis and Religious Experience*, New Haven, CT: Yale University Press.

[41] Kanter 2000 p. 254.

MY SQUIGGLE. HIS MODIFICATION. HIS COMMENT — ENGLAND.

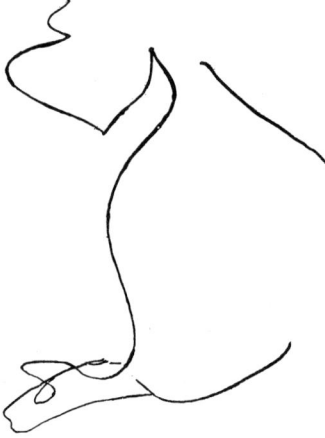

HIS SQUIGGLE. MY MODIFICATION. HIS COMMENT — A FISH.

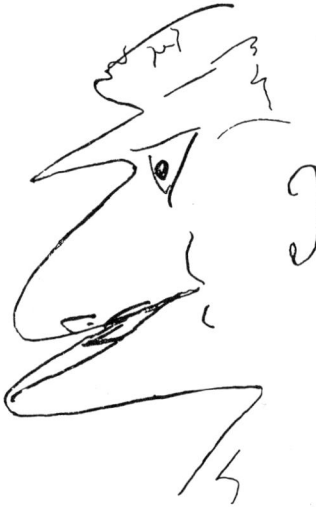

MY SQUIGGLE. HIS MODIFICATION. HIS COMMENT — A SEA LION WITH A BABY.

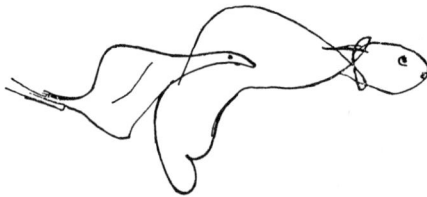

Fig. 10.1 Squiggles.

Meanwhile, with his child patients, Winnicott used a game in which, just as he said the mother brings her baby's dreams and illusions into being through providing a "simplified bit of the world",[42] he did the same for his child patients. He would squiggle a line for them, ask them to complete it, and then squiggle a line for him. An example was a 9-year-old boy, Philip, expelled from prep school on account of stealing. Describing his case, Winnicott showed how, through Philip's free associations to their squiggles together (see Fig. 10.1), Philip was able to confront and deal with fears and nightmares contributing to his problems at school thereby enabling him to return and do well.[43]

But what about religion? Winnicott told the Jungian analyst, Michael Fordham, that whenever his detractors accused him of being irreligious, it "always turned out that what they were annoyed about was that I was not myself religious in their own particular way".[44] Subsequently he came to locate the source of religious experience in the silence and stillness of being alone. He linked it with the solitude of sexual partners with each other after making love. He also linked it with the solitude of babies in the presence of their mothers.

He described how, through pregnancy and the early weeks of her baby's life, "a state of heightened sensitivity", a "normal illness" of oneness, of "maternal preoccupation", develops in the mother. It is this, he said, that enables her to "feel herself into her infant's place, and so meet her infant's needs",[45] thereby protecting his "going on being" from inner and outer impingement. Through meeting his needs the mother transforms and enriches the baby's illusions and dreams with reality. He can thereby bear "to become unintegrated, to flounder. He can bear to be in a state in which there is no orientation".[46] Neither active action, nor passive reaction. Alone in her presence. Having taken her care into him, he can begin also to bear being alone without her. We learn of this aloneness in the togetherness of making love when afterwards, if all goes well, said Winnicott, "each partner is alone and is contented to be alone . . . sharing solitude . . . relatively free from the property that we call 'withdrawal'".[47]

Winnicott related this to religion. He spoke about the "withdrawal into a personal inner world" of the mystic for whom, he maintained, "loss of contact

---

[42] Winnicott 1945 p. 153.

[43] D. W. Winnicott (1953) Symptom tolerance in paediatrics, in Winnicott 1958 pp. 101–17, 109.

[44] To Michael Fordham, 11 June 1954, in Winnicott 1987 p. 74.

[45] D. W. Winnicott (1956) Primary maternal preoccupation, in Winnicott 1958 pp. 300–305, 302, 303, 304.

[46] D. W. Winnicott (1958) The capacity to be alone, in Winnicott 1965 pp. 29–36, 34.

[47] Ibid. p. 31.

with the world of shared reality . . . [is] counterbalanced by a gain in terms of feeling real".[48] In health there is a "core" of the personality, corresponding to the true part of the divided true-false self, which, he claimed, we know must never be communicated with, met with, or influenced from outside. It is the aspect of us, he said, which, at heart, we know makes us each "an isolate, permanently non-communicating, permanently unknown, in fact unfound".[49] It is an area where "quietude is linked with stillness . . . for ever immune from the reality principle, and for ever silent . . . like the music of the spheres, absolutely personal".[50] It is from here, he maintained, that we find the oneness of inner and outer, subject and object, of language, culture, and religion.

Winnicott also wrote of the baby's initial ruthlessness in treating his mother as though she were one with his imagined idea of her. The potential space between inner and outer can only open up, he said, and the baby can only begin to feel concern for his mother as someone separate from himself, provided she survives his ruthless destructiveness and gives him opportunities to repair its effects.[51] The same too is true of therapy.

An example was a 2-year-old girl, Gabrielle, whom Winnicott saw occasionally as a patient. At first she related to him as if he were the same as her imagined idea of her baby sister, greedily wanting to eat her up and have their mother to herself. Through Winnicott surviving her destructiveness she came to recognize that he was not one with her fantasies about him. She became able to use the potential, overlapping, subject–object space thereby opened up to explore her destructiveness. It enabled her also to explore other feelings and ideas, including differences between them about religion. Of the ending of one of their last meetings together, when she was 4, Winnicott wrote:

> She had now practically finished with the toys and said to me: "Do you go to church?" I didn't know what to answer.
> *Me*: Well, sometimes. Do you?
> *Gabrielle*: I would like to go, but mummy and daddy would not like to. I don't know why.
> *Me*: Why do people go to church?
> *Gabrielle*: I don't know.
> *Me*: Is it something to do with God?
> Gabrielle: No.[52]

---

48 D. W. Winnicott (1963) Communicating and not communicating leading to a study of certain opposites, in Winnicott 1965 pp. 179–92, 185–6.

49 Ibid. p. 187.

50 Ibid. pp. 190, 192.

51 D. W. Winnicott (1963) The development of the capacity for concern, in Winnicott 1965 pp. 73–82.

52 D. W. Winnicott (1977) *The Piggle*, London: Penguin, 1980 p. 182.

At their next meeting she made a pipe-cleaner figure to represent Winnicott. She twisted it till, she said, he was all gone. "So the Winnicott you invented," he said, "was all yours and he's now finished with, and no one else can ever have him".[53]

Winnicott spoke more about the child and adult patient's movement from an illusion of oneness with the mother or analyst to recognition of separateness between them in a talk he gave in New York in November 1968. He described the illusion of oneness with another as "object-relating", and the illusion of oneness with another recognized to be separate from oneself as "object-usage".[54] Enabling the patient to move from one to the other might involve the analyst, like the "good enough" mother, providing physical and emotional support for his patients so that they can then begin to use him and his interpretations as separate from them.

Perhaps it was the fact that, in this, he advocated departing from the reliance of orthodox psychoanalysis on talking as means of therapy that contributed to his New York lecture not being very well received. Whatever the reason, it was followed by his suffering a massive heart attack in his hotel. But he recovered and returned to London. The next year he gave a talk to Anglican priests. He advised them that if someone asked for their help but was boring then they needed psychiatric treatment whereas, he said, "if he sustains your interest, no matter how grave his distress and conflict, then you can help him all right."[55] He emphasized the un-boring liveliness of the psyche as the essence of health, and, as for the healing essence of therapy, he emphasized "Faith in human nature".[56] He also emphasized playing – highlighting its importance with italics:

> *Psychotherapy has to do with two people playing together. The corollary of this is that where playing is not possible then the work done by the therapist is directed towards bringing the patient from a state of not being able to play into a state of being able to play.*[57]

But this was published posthumously. After watching TV one evening with Clare, sitting on the floor, as they often did together, they fell asleep, and in the early hours of 25 January 1971, she discovered him dead beside her, his head snuggled into his armchair.

Winnicott today: Christopher Bollas

Winnicott's work is still enormously endearing. Too endearing, some might say. For, although he addressed hate, and criticized Jung's neglect of destructiveness

[53] Ibid. p. 189.

[54] D. W. Winnicott (1969) The use of an object, in Winnicott 1971 pp. 101–11, 110.

[55] In Phillips p. 25.

[56] D. W. Winnicott (1970) Early one morning, *Case Conference*, **16** pp. 504–5.

[57] D. W. Winnicott (1971) Playing: A theoretical statement, in Winnicott 1971 pp. 44–61, 44.

(see p. 92), he seems to have found it hard to address the destructiveness of his patients.[58] In this, it seems, Winnicott was akin to the mind-cure and Christian Science therapists William James criticized for being over-optimistic in emphasizing goodness and love to the neglect of badness and hate.

But, like William James, Winnicott, as we have seen, also related therapy to religion. So too do his followers. After his death Marion Milner noted that when she read in a religious book that "to discover God as myself is also to discover Him as other than myself" she was reminded of Winnicott's idea of what she called a "two-way journey" towards finding the objective reality of both object and subject in the space in between.[59]

Subsequently some, as I have indicated, have related Winnicott's version of psychoanalysis to Catholicism.[60] Others relate it to Buddhism. Still others relate his work to religion more generally.[61] Particularly appealing and widely read in this respect is the work of the US-born, London-based psychoanalyst, Christopher Bollas. Just as Winnicott said psychoanalysis both uses play and seeks to enable its patients to play, Bollas says that it both uses free association and seeks to enable its patients to free associate. The aim and method of psychoanalysis are the same – free association playing. Like Winnicott, Bollas also argues that to accomplish this the analyst should enable the patient to use him as a me/not-me transitional object. Bollas puts this in terms of the analyst enabling the patient to use him as a "transformational object" so that the uniqueness of the patient's spirit – his "idiom" or "character", as Bollas puts it – can come into being.

Bollas also argues that, if the patient is to be able to use the analyst as his transitional or transformational object, the analyst must be psychologically one with his patient, just as Winnicott claimed that the "good enough" mother is initially psychologically one with her baby. It entails, says Bollas, recovering the oneness of analyst and patient recommended by Freud in advocating that analysts adopt an attitude of "evenly-suspended attention" free from all censorship and selection so as "to catch the drift of the patient's unconscious with his own unconscious".[62]

....

[58] Hopkins.

[59] M. Milner (1972) Winnicott and the two-way journey, in M. Milner (1987) *The Suppressed Madness of Sane Men*, London: Routledge, pp. 246–52, 151.

[60] Meissner, see also Kristeva in Chapter 12 below.

[61] See, for example, J. Jones (1991) *Contemporary Psychoanalysis and Religion: Transference and Transcendence*, New Haven, CT: Yale University Press; D. M. Wulff (1997) *Psychology of Religion*, New York: Wiley; M. Eigen (1998) *The Psychoanalytic Mystic*, London: Free Association Books; A. Molino (1999) *The Couch and the Tree*, London: Constable.

[62] S. Freud (1912e) Recommendations to physicians practising psycho-analysis, **SE12** pp. 111–20, 111; S. Freud (1923) Two encyclopaedia articles, **SE18** pp. 235–59, 239, see p. 53 above.

Much more than Freud and Winnicott, however, Bollas puts the transforming effect of the oneness of the analyst's unconscious with that of the patient, or the transitional or transformational oneness of me and not-me in terms of religion:

> The Old Testament describes how God spoke inside the body and mind of the other . . . hallucinating hysterics of the Middle Ages heard the voices of the devil in their ears . . . female spiritualists [in the nineteenth century] acted as mediums for the voices of the departed . . . [similarly] the analyst who receives the transferences willingly, and who quietly notes the many moods, self states, wild ideas and credible theories that occur inside him, gradually comes to the place of two-in-one.[63]

Through putting into words the free associations mobilized in, and through his unconscious being "two-in-one" with that of his patient, says Bollas, the analyst punctures and destabilizes the patient's frozen account of himself, which often constitutes both his adaptation against trauma and the unhappiness for which he seeks help. Through oneness with the patient the analyst seeks to enliven and transform the patient's rigidified soul or spirit into fluidity. In this Bollas likens the work of the analyst to that of the poet described by Shakespeare in *A Midsummer Night's Dream*

> as imagination bodies forth
> The form of things unknown, the poet's pen
> Turns them to shapes, and gives to aery nothing
> A local habitation a name.[64]

In analysis this transformation depends, says Bollas, again drawing on Winnicott's writing, on the oneness of the patient's "multiple uses of the analyst's personality".[65] The patient can thereby come to what Bollas calls the "unthought known".[66] He relates it to God:

> What is the intelligence that moves through the mind to create its objects, to shape its inscapes, to word itself, to gather moods, to effect the other's arriving ideas, to . . . to . . . to? If there is a God this is where it lives [in the unconscious], a mystery working itself through the materials of life, giving us shape and passing us on to others.[67]

In thus bringing psychoanalysis together with religion, Bollas, like many other psychoanalysts and psychotherapists, draws not only on the work of Winnicott but on that of Bion who, as we will see, drew in his final work on religious and mystical writing.

---

63 C. Bollas (1999) *The Mystery of Things*, London: Routledge, p. 21.

64 Ibid. p. 126.

65 Ibid. p. 192.

66 C. Bollas (1987) *The Shadow of the Object*, London: Free Association Books.

67 Bollas 1999 p. 195.

Chapter 11

Wilfred Bion

Transforming at-one-ment

Wilfred Bion was no enthusiast for conventional religion. He dismissed his paternal grandfather as "some sort of missionary in India", and his mother's family as "probably missionary or 'off' missionary in the sense that builders and decorators talk about 'off' white".[1] He described the inhibiting effects of experiencing his father as a fierce "Arf, Arfer" – figure modelled on the "Our Father" of the Lord's Prayer. He despised the use of religion by his boarding school to justify its repression of sex. He was also scathing about groups and organizations sanctifying their leaders or insightful members as gods or saints.

Nevertheless Bion very much allied psychoanalysis with religious or mystical "at-one-ment" with what he called "O" or "ultimate reality" as a means of transforming the formlessness contributing to the upsets bringing people into analysis into something that can be known. I will seek to explain this after detailing his insights about psychosis, and the love arguably inspiring them. I will begin, however, with fears initially obstructing his at-one-ment with others.

Fearfulness

Born on 8 September 1897 in Muttra in the North West Provinces of India, Bion dwelt in old age on how, unlike his father, who was a big game hunter, he was a "sniveller who was frightened even by the sight of a tiger trap".[2] He recounted his fear of what other boys might think stopping him showing his tears on first arriving at boarding school when he was eight. Later fear made him hide his sexual feelings for one of his best friends lest he upset him. He was fearful of being treated as a coward for not going to war, and upset when the recruiting officer dismissed him as a mere schoolboy. It was only through his father's influence, he said, that he was recruited for officer training (in 1916), after which he went the next year with his tank battalion to Belgium.

---

[1] To Francesca, 1 April 1951, in W. R. Bion (1985) *All My Sins Remembered* and *The Other Side of Genius*, Abingdon: Fleetwood Press, p. 79.

[2] W. R. Bion (1982) *The Long Week-End*, London: Free Association Books, p. 32.

Later he told his parents what he could not tell them at the time. He described the mud, muddle, and confusion, and his senior officers' determination to find heroes and get him awarded the Victoria Cross for his part in the Battle of Ypres, despite his feeling himself to be an utter coward. "I was so terrified that I would run away," he later wrote, "I could hardly think of anything else".[3] Back home on leave he hated himself for being so preoccupied with fear of the war he could not be at one with his mother. Defeated by his "taciturn moroseness," he wrote, she tried joking:

[She] asked if I knew the riddle of the miser's most hated flower. "It's the anemone," she said, "because it reminds him of someone asking 'Any money? Any money?' " My response was a stony silence which was so hostile that it frightened me.[4]

Only by overcoming his fears – most of all his fear of death – did he gain courage to face what was going on:

I wasn't interested in religion or world politics or any rot like that. I was merely an insignificant scrap of humanity that was being intolerably persecuted by unknown powers, and I was going to score off those powers by dying . . . . With this new idea before me, I felt better. I didn't feel afraid any more.[5]

Doing away with his fear emboldened him. It enabled him to encourage his men from the top of one of the trenches: "I must have been very nearly mad to do it," he admitted. "But I never *thought* more clearly in my life".[6]

Fear could still stop him thinking or knowing, in the Battle of Amiens, on 8 August 1918, for instance. Frightened at not being able to see and mistaking what he did see because of mist and the smoke of enemy fire, he found himself crouching against it with a runner, Sweeting. And then, he said,

A shell burst on top of us, and I heard a groan from Sweeting. The left side of his tunic seemed covered with blood, and as I looked, I discovered that the whole of his left side had been torn away so that the inside of the trunk lay exposed. But he was not dead . . . . I pretended to bandage him, but of course the field dressing was far too small and simply didn't come near to covering the cavity. He kept on saying, "I'm done for, sir! I'm done for!", hoping against hope I would contradict him . . . . He kept trying to cough, but of course the wind only came out of his side. He kept asking me why he couldn't cough.[7]

---

[3] W. R. Bion (1991) *A Memoir of the Future*, London: Karnac, p. 455.

[4] Bion 1982 p. 190.

[5] W. R. Bion (1997) *War Memoirs 1917–1919*, London: Karnac, pp. 94–5.

[6] Ibid. p. 106.

[7] Ibid. pp. 124 127.

Fearful of facing the horror at the time, it returned to plague him as a night-mare when he was in London on leave from France:

> "Mother, Mother . . . You will write to my mother sir, won't you?"
> "No, blast you, I shan't! Shut up! Can't you see I don't want to be disturbed?"[8]

Back in France he again found himself "paralyzed at the thought of action". Fear stopped him thinking, "my brain would *not* work . . . unable to shake off a kind of sluggishness and terror that threatened to crush all life out of me".[9] Added to that was grief at the death of friends in battle, "love had died. Love for anyone and anything . . . I could never flame with life again after James, Ernest, Charles and I were extinguished at Cambrai".[10]

After the war he went to Queen's College, Oxford, to study history, spent a year after graduating in Poitiers, and then returned to teach at his old school. But he was dismissed, as he later understood it, for not having the courage to stand up for himself against the mother of one of his pupils falsely accusing him of abusing her son. To this was added the hurt of no sooner becoming engaged to his friend's sister than she jilted him for another man because, Bion surmised, he was not the courageous hero she had expected him to be. Dejected, he went into therapy. He also decided to become a therapist himself and to this end, studied medicine at University College London.

He qualified in 1930 and not long after began work at the Tavistock Clinic, where his patients included Samuel Beckett. He went with him to Jung's 1935 Tavistock Clinic lectures at which Bion's therapist, Hadfield, persuaded Jung to detail his method of active imagination, involving asking patients to attend to whatever images happens to occur to them. A couple of years later, in 1937, Bion went into analysis with a Quaker, John Rickman. Subsequently, following the death of his mother (in early 1939), Bion met an actress, Betty Jardine, who became his first wife. They married in April 1940. The same year Bion's first published article appeared. It was about enemies deflecting their opponent's attention through propaganda aimed at arousing their imagined fears. The answer, said Bion, lies in allaying such fears by mobilizing people to join together in civil defence aimed at dealing with the actuality of danger.[11]

He applied the same idea as an army psychiatrist assessing men for officer training through observing their capacity to subordinate their individual fears

---

[8] Bion 1982 p. 264.

[9] Bion 1997 p. 156 – Bion's emphasis.

[10] Ibid. p. 150.

[11] W. R. Bion (1940) The "war of nerves", in E. Miller (ed.) *The Neuroses of War*, London: Macmillan, pp. 180–200.

to the common cause of seeking to solve a task assigned to them as a group. Bion pursued a similar method with Rickman in seeking to rehabilitate men psychiatrically incapacitated from military service. Bion and Rickman sought to enable them to face together their psychiatric difficulties, through meeting collectively each day to discuss what was going on between them on the wing of the hospital where they were being treated. As a result morale on the wing significantly improved. But the experiment was soon stopped. Bion returned to officer selection and, after the Allied landings in France, he was posted to help with psychiatric rehabilitation there.

It was in France, in Normandy, that he learnt of the birth of his daughter, Parthenope (on 17 February 1945), followed almost immediately by the death of her mother, Betty, from septicaemia or a pulmonary embolism. Bion was devastated. He returned to England and after the war, moved to Iver Heath, near Slough, with a family – the Ransoms – who had looked after Parthenope during the war. Now misery at the loss of Betty closed him from oneness with her. It culminated in an incident in which she called to him to come to her in the garden and, despite her mounting distress, he refused to budge.

> I felt as if I were gripped in a vice. No. I would *not* go. At last the nurse, having glanced at me with astonishment, got up ignoring my prohibition, and fetched her. The spell snapped. I was released. The baby had stopped weeping and was being comforted by maternal arms. But I, I had lost my child.[12]

Shocked by being so blocked off by grief from attending to her, he went into analysis, this time with Melanie Klein.

He also resumed work at the Tavistock Clinic, where he pioneered group therapy. It involved trying to persuade patients to tackle their problems collectively by attending to what went on psychologically between them as a group. He called the psychological data thereby emerging, "proto-mental" phenomena.[13] They surfaced, he said, in feelings of fear, security, depression, or sex, diverting them from attending to what was actually going on psychologically between them. Instead they looked dependently to him to become their God-like leader, or to someone else to fight or take flight from, or to a couple to make something new.

Bion likened women and men attending to what actually goes on to Freud's account of consciousness coming into being on discovering that wishful thinking does not bring about what one wishes or wants unless one takes

---

[12] Bion 1985 p. 70.

[13] W. R. Bion (1950) Experiences in groups, *Human Relations*, 3(1) pp. 3–14, in W. R. Bion (1961) *Experiences in Groups*, London: Tavistock, pp. 93–114, 101.

account of reality. With this discovery, beginning in early infancy, wrote Freud,[14] attention and means of mentally registering its findings come into being. Thinking thereby becomes possible as an intermediary between wishing, seeing, and doing.

But as Bion had often noticed in his own case, attention can also be obstructed by fear. Now he put this in terms of Klein's account of young children being so fearful of what their curiosity might lead them to discover in their mother's body they dare not pursue it by attending to, or being curious about what happens around them.[15] Bion likened the object of this fear to the disaster befalling Oedipus on seeking to discover the truth about himself and thereby learning that he had murdered his father and married his mother. Bion wrote about this in articles published between 1948 and 1951. He also wrote about his analysis of a man who avoided attending to what was going on between himself and others by treating them as an "imaginary twin" of himself.[16] Bion's account of this case, in November 1950, qualified him for membership of the BPAS.

Bion in love

Soon after becoming a member of the BPAS Bion fell in love with a young widow, Francesca McCallum. He first caught sight of her in the dining room of the Tavistock Clinic where she was working as a research assistant. She was 28. Being terribly formal, she later wrote, he got a colleague to introduce them. Soon after they first went out together, Bion pictured her to himself in a letter he wrote to her in the early hours of that Good Friday.

> Francesca dear, This does not seem a very sensible time in the morning to start writing you a letter but then I feel I cannot wait till tomorrow . . . I walked back with a great wind blowing hazy clouds across a moon which was never visible but made all the trees stand out a deep grey against the silvery meadows and water. And all the time I could see you, and still see you, looking more ravishingly beautiful, as you did all the evening when I was with you, than anyone could believe possible.[17]

On Easter Sunday he wrote to her about finishing "a contribution to a book edited by Roger Money-Kyrle".[18] In it he quoted Freud's account of the emergence from pleasure and pain into consciousness of what our senses tell us about outer

---

[14] S. Freud (1911) Formulations on the two principles of mental functioning, SE12 pp. 218–26.

[15] W. R. Bion (1952) Group dynamics, in Bion 1961 pp. 141–91.

[16] W. R. Bion (1950) The imaginary twin, in W. R. Bion (1967) *Second Thoughts*, London: Heinemann, pp. 3–22.

[17] To Francesca, 22 March 1951, in Bion 1985 p. 73.

[18] To Francesca, 24 March 1951, ibid. p. 75.

reality.[19] Bion described this awareness being attacked in madness, as in the case of a patient who, cutting off one sentence from the next with four or five minute gaps in between, said:

> "I have a problem I am trying to work out."
> "As a child I never had phantasies."
> "I knew they weren't facts so I stopped them."
> "I don't dream nowadays."[20]

After another pause he added, in a bewildered tone of voice, "I don't know what to do now". Bion commented, "About a year ago you told me you were no good at thinking. Just now you said you were working out a problem – obviously something you were thinking about." "Yes," said the patient. To this Bion said:

> But you went on with the thought that you had no phantasies in childhood; and then that you had no dreams; you then said that you did not know what to do. It must mean that without phantasies and without dreams you have not the means with which to think out your problem.[21]

The patient might not be able to dream. Inspired by love of Francesca, Bion had no such difficulty. He wrote to her about his own and his 6-year-old daughter's dreams. "Francesca my darling," he wrote, "This is only a note to say I love you". He went on to say how Parthenope had woken up in the night with a nightmare, adding:

> How people can think of childhood as "happy"' I do not know. A horrible bogey-ridden, demon-haunted time it was to me and then one has not the fortitude, or callosities perhaps, with which to deal with it.[22]

He ended with his own dreaming: "It takes me an enormous time to write these letters because I stop at every other word to think about you, or I should say to dream about you."[23]

The next day he wrote to her about going to Gian-Carlo Menotti's opera, *The Consul*, first staged in London the previous month. The opera, said Bion, was:

> An immensely moving experience and what added to the depth of my happiness was the knowledge that but for you I would not have had it. Your presence pours a soft radiance of joy over my life.[24]

....

[19] Freud 1911. See also P. Talamo (1997) Bion: A Freudian innovator, *British Journal of Psychotherapy*, **14** pp. 47–59.

[20] W. R. Bion (1955) Language and the schizophrenic, in M. Klein, P. Heimann and R.E. Money-Kyrle (eds) *New Directions in Psycho-Analysis*, London: Tavistock, pp. 220–39, 227.

[21] Ibid. p. 227.

[22] To Francesca, 28 March 1951, Bion 1985 p. 76.

[23] Ibid. p. 76.

[24] To Francesca, 29 March 1951, ibid. p. 77.

And then he again returned to his dream pictures of her:

> Darling Francesca: I have just been in a day dream again thinking with longing of your dear presence. I find that quite trivial moments seem fixed deep in my heart; for some reason moments such as one when, after I went to look for a taxi when we came out of Kettner's, I looked back and saw you standing waiting in the distance under the theatre. There seems no reason why one particular moment like that should be so clear to my sight but so it is.[25]

He wrote of the thrill of seeing her in his "mind's eye".[26] He wrote of his thankfulness about daring to risk falling in love, and about their decision to marry.

> Francesca, my darling . . . I am more thankful than I can say that something gave me the courage to know that when I found that you had become the first person in my heart, that was the right and proper foundation without which one would build in vain, no matter what one tried to do. . . . Darling Francesca, without you I am nothing. "Sorrow follows folly as the berries grow on holly and – / Oh! 'tis folly – to be afraid of love'.[27]

He wrote of her inspiring his work. "Dear Sweetheart . . . my work is coming alive; the dull numb mechanical routine into which I have fallen is bursting wide open and it is all you my darling, my darling Francesca".[28] He also wrote of her bringing back to life his feelings for Parthenope:

> You have given Parthenope back to me and made me feel what it is like to have a child. You cannot think how terrible it has been to feel all the time that every day she was becoming more lost to me till at times she hardly seemed my child at all.[29]

He told her how their colleagues – Bowlby, Sutherland, and others – congratulated him on their engagement. Perhaps thinking about the house, Redcourt, in Croydon that they were getting ready as a home together, he wrote: "whereas before (Before Francesca) even one late night a week left me tired out by the week-end, now tonight I feel as fresh as paint".[30] She brought him awake. "My darling," he wrote, "Even my crusted and hardened armour plate of fossilized worry seems to be shaling off each time I see you".[31] Awake and dreaming. "Francesca darling," he wrote on 3 May 1951, "if this is a dream it is the longest

[25] To Francesca, 1 April 1951, ibid. p. 80.

[26] To Francesca, undated, ibid. p. 81.

[27] To Francesca, 6 April 1951, ibid. pp. 81–2.

[28] To Francesca, 10 April 1951, ibid. p. 84.

[29] To Francesca, 11 April 1951, ibid. p. 85.

[30] To Francesca, 13 April 1951, ibid. p. 86.

[31] To Francesca, 29 April 1951, ibid. p. 93.

and most marvellous dream I have ever had; if it is not a dream, then I don't know how to contain myself".[32]

They married on 9 June 1951. Following a reception at Brown's Hotel, and postponing taking a honeymoon together (which turned out not to be possible till the summer of 1958 when they went to Paris together for a week), Francesca sought to get to know Parthenope better. She went away with her for a fortnight to Bournemouth. Bion wrote letters to Francesca there sometimes several times a day. In a third letter one day he mused on a phone call with her inspiring his work:

> My darling Wife, The sound of your dear voice has really put some life into me in a most magical way . . . It has even had the effect of making me get out my own group [group dynamics-1952] paper and look at it. . . . The other paper I spoke about was an expansion of my [imaginary twin-1950] membership paper.[33]

Bion again wrote of how she inspired his work when, a year later, she was in hospital after giving birth to their first child, Julian (on 30 July 1952):

> Francesca my darling . . . I had the best session yet with my problem child and although there were extraneous reasons for it, it is also a sign of good work here. My darling sweetheart this is all you. If it were not for the thought of your love for me I don't believe I could cure anybody or anything.[34]

Two years later Francesca gave birth to their second child, Nicola (on 13 June 1955). This was followed by more letters at the end of the next month from that year's psychoanalytic congress in Geneva, where he talked about applying Klein's ideas in analysing psychosis.

Analyzing psychosis

In his Geneva talk, and perhaps thinking more about his waking dreaming about Francesca, Bion again described the lack of such dreaming in schizophrenia. Attacking conscious awareness, he said, the schizophrenic gets rid of the resulting fragments. He then feels both imprisoned in his mind and at the same time attacked by its ejected fragments as "bizarre objects" attacking him from outside. He lives in a world not of dreams but of things which he cannot integrate but can only "agglomerate or compress".[35]

---

[32] To Francesa, 3 May 1951, ibid. p. 95.

[33] To Francesca, 9 July 1951, ibid. pp. 104–5.

[34] To Francesca, 14 August 1952, ibid. p. 110.

[35] W. R. Bion (1956) Development of schizophrenic thought, *IJPA*, **37** pp. 344–6, in Bion 1987 pp. 36–42, 41.

Bion gave examples of the way, in psychosis, patients get rid of sensations as if they were things through convulsively jerking their bodies,[36] or through depositing what they take in with their eyes onto walls and into corners of the room to become visual hallucinations.[37] They attack any link with the analyst taking in and making what they experience bearable.[38] In such states of mind, Bion speculated,[39] linking one notion with another so much evokes the possibility and envy of a couple making love that the patient hates and destroys it even as an idea. Bion sent this paper off for publication in mid-December 1958. Soon after he wrote numerous notes about analysing psychotic patients which, after his death, Francesca arranged to have published as a book.

The resulting collection, *Cogitations*, begins with what the mathematician, Henri Poincaré, described as the transforming effect of a "selected fact". '[It] must unite elements long since known, but till then scattered and seemingly foreign to each other, and suddenly introduce order where the appearance of disorder reigned.'[40] Bion described sensory facts – "touch and smell" – coming together in "love-making".[41] By contrast psychoanalysis brings together non-sensory, psychological facts.

He went on to describe the analyst interpreting to the patient what is going on between them as also involving what Poincaré called bringing together "elements long since known . . . scattered and seemingly foreign to each other".[42] If, said Bion, the analyst can tolerate what Klein called the depression involved in bringing together good and bad he can interpret what goes on between him and the patient so as to "introduce order into this complexity and so make it accessible".[43] The analyst's job is to help the patient by selecting the unifying fact. This involves the analyst in translating the data he observes into an idea. If he does this lovingly, wrote Bion, it leads to understanding, "if carried out violently . . . with hate, then it leads to splitting and to cruel juxtaposition or fusion."[44]

Early the next month, on his way from Croydon to his Harley Street consulting room, Bion fainted in Victoria Station. He was taken for tests to St George's

[36] W. R. Bion (1957) Differentiation of the psychotic from the non-psychotic personalities, *IJPA*, **38** pp. 266–75.

[37] W. R. Bion (1958) On hallucination, *IJPA*, **39** pp. 341–9.

[38] W. R. Bion (1958) On arrogance, *IJPA*, **39** pp. 144–6.

[39] W. R. Bion (1959) Attacks on linking, *IJPA*, **40** pp. 308–15.

[40] 10 January 1959, in W. R. Bion (1992) *Cogitations*, London: Karnac, p. 2.

[41] Ibid. pp. 4, 5.

[42] Ibid. p. 5.

[43] Ibid. p. 5.

[44] 10 January 1959, ibid. p. 22.

LETTERS TO THE CHILDREN

It was lovely to have the oranges from you. I like oranges very much but they are nicer because you were so kind to send them. When they dust the room here they turn a handle on the bed and this makes wheels come down so they can push the bed with me in it and I have a fine ride to the other side of the room. They call the rooms here wards. Then a very nice fat lady comes and pushes a big thing that looks like an enormous iron cake. This whirls round and polishes the floor making a lovely noise as if you were being chased by a motor bus. You can see the lady likes doing it very much indeed. And it stops sick people thinking about their illness because they are thinking what that lovely noise can be.

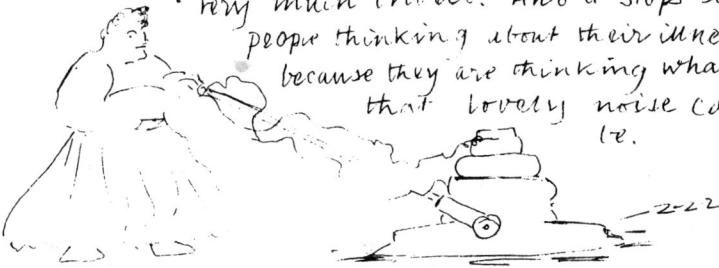

Goodbye my dear I hope I shall come back and see you all soon. With love from Daddy.

Fig. 11.1 Letter to his children.

Hospital, from where he sent his children a drawing (see Fig. 11.1 above) of the cleaning lady on the ward together with a letter describing her:

> A very nice fat lady comes and pushes a big thing that looks like an enormous iron cake. This whirls round and polishes the floor making a lovely noise as if you were being chased by a motor bus. You can see the lady likes doing it very much indeed. And it stops sick people thinking about their illness because they are thinking what that lovely noise can be.[45]

---

[45] Letters to the children, 1959, in Bion 1985 p. 169.

He also wrote to Francesca:

> My darling, It really did seem as if the sunshine had gone out of the ward when you
> went out just then, but thanks to letters I can start writing straight away. It is a queer
> thing about love that it teaches you that certain common phrases which seem never to
> have much meaning are really quite true. If it weren't for you I would not have found
> that out about the sunshine.[46]

The next day, he wrote, "My darling . . . I continue to cogitate on my paper
["Attacks on linking"] but it is a curiously elusive subject".[47] "Like you I feel
only half alive though I hardly realize it till I become wholly alive through your
letter", he went on, "as I write to you I feel I want to be writing a marvellous
paper".[48] And on the following day,

> I *know* you love me: and that is all I want or need to know. I *know* you are by my side
> in thought and would be so in fact if it were wise to be here rather than somewhere
> else. I *know* we must both be troubled and depressed and faint-hearted at times, or we
> would not be human. . . . I am wondering whether I ought to take the chance of look-
> ing at all that group stuff. I believe it might be very well worth while and it could be
> the start of a useful piece of work.[49]

Inspired by Francesca he got together his "group stuff". It was published as a
book, *Experiences in Groups*. Meanwhile, and also perhaps inspired by the pictures and dreams awoken in him by love of Francesca and their children, he
innovatively took issue with Freud. He noted how Freud described dream-
work as the means by which unconscious material is transformed into the
manifest dream we consciously attend to in recalling it. Bion now argued the
reverse. Conscious attention, he said, comes first: "conscious material has to be
subjected to dream-work," he wrote, "to render it fit for storing, selection, and
suitable for transformation" into the stuff of memory, conscious and unconscious.[50] Without dream-work, he added, the data of inner and outer reality
are not available for learning from experience. "In this sense," he went on, "the
dream seems to play a part in the mental life of the individual which is ana-
logous to the digestive process in the alimentary life of the individual."[51]

Around the same time Bion noted, as he had in an essay, "On arrogance",[52]
that attacking linking or pairing of one thing with another includes taking

46 To Francesca, 4 February 1959, ibid. pp. 124–5.

47 To Francesca, 5 February 1959, ibid. p. 125.

48 To Francesca, 6 February 1959, ibid. pp. 125–6.

49 To Francesca, 7 February 1959, ibid. p. 128.

50 27 July 1959, Bion 1992 p. 43.

51 28 July 1959, ibid. p. 45.

52 Bion 1958 (see note 38 above).

back into the self a superego that harshly attacks all links with others, including the fantasy of expelling and projecting things into them.[53] He also noted the intolerance of frustration contributing to psychotic hatred of reality. Exploring ideas he had developed in the essay about which he had written in one of his first love letters to Francesca, he suggested this hatred contributes to psychotic inability to dream. Calling dreaming "reverie" and "alpha", he wrote:

> In the psychotic we find no capacity for reverie, no alpha, or a very deficient alpha, and so none of the capacities – or extremely macilent [lean] capacities – which depend on alpha, namely attention, passing of judgement, memory, and dream-pictures, or pictorial imagery that is capable of yielding associations.[54]

Rather than dream, one patient "winces at each word", said Bion, to get rid of them as if they were projectiles to be evacuated.[55] Lacking associations, Bion observed, words in psychosis function like pure notes in music, "devoid of undertones or overtones".[56] The psychotic may rid himself of experience with a "grimace of pain" or "elbow-rubbing".[57] Perhaps thinking of his children, Bion noted how the child makes conscious material unconscious in learning to walk so as to make it available for "unconscious waking thinking".[58] The psychotic does away with all such thinking and dreaming.

To avoid confusion with Freud's quite different account of dreaming, Bion called the dreaming he believed to be crucial to consciousness "attention".[59] Without wide-awake attention and dreaming, Bion went on, the psychotic's tears have no depth, his jolliness no friendliness, his hate is in bits. There is nothing but "a labile façade".[60] Following Descartes' dictum, *cogito ergo sum* [I think therefore I am], Bion concluded that, in attacking thinking, the personality in psychosis "ceases to exist".[61] In attacking thinking, the psychotic may stammer as means to "an evacuation of awareness of what is currently taking place".[62] Another patient, a widower, stood up, pointed, and said, "My wife, it's my wife! She's coming for

---

53 E.g. undated note, Bion 1992 p. 35.

54 5 August 1959, ibid. p. 53.

55 6 August 1959, ibid. p. 55.

56 10 August 1959, ibid. p. 63.

57 10 August 1959, ibid. p. 64.

58 8 September 1959, ibid. p. 71.

59 12 September 1959, ibid. p. 73.

60 13 September 1959, ibid. p. 74.

61 19 September 1959, ibid. p. 76.

62 19 September 1959, ibid. p. 77.

me! Stop her!" [63] Thus exclaiming, wrote Bion, the patient evacuated an undigested visual image of his dead wife, through his eyes. A couple of weeks later, at the end of October 1959, Bion wrote of this or another patient:

> It's hard to recall anything the patient said. Instead splitting into a mass of tiny persecutory depressions: the door slams; singing in his head; a pain in his ankle: "I don't know why; I'm sorry; the waitress brought some coffee; only half a cup"; and – despairingly, "*I could not go on*" . . . "undigested" fragments, i.e. not proper pictorial images but facts sensually perceived yet remaining as bits of sensory awareness. [64]

Faced with such fragments, what is the analyst to do? In his love letters to Francesca, Bion had written about dreaming. Now he again wrote about dreaming. Analysts, he wrote, must "dream" the session so as to make the psychological data involved available to consciousness. And this means having enough sleep to do this and still stay awake. [65] In a note on St Valentine's Day, 1960, he also emphasized our inborn "capacity for love". [66] He described the baby's initial pleasure in "proto-real objects felt to be real and alive" while converting pain into "dead objects destroyed by its hate". [67]

He reiterated his earlier observations about attention "as 'dreaming' what is going on". [68] He compared the analyst dreaming and thereby giving form to what goes on between him and his patient to the work of the scientist and artist, of whom he wrote:

> He is someone who is able to digest facts, i.e. sense data, and then to present the digested facts, my alpha-elements, in a way that makes it possible for the weak assimilators to go on from there. Thus the artist helps the non-artist to digest, say, the Little Street in Delft by doing alpha-work on his sense impressions and "publishing" the result so that others who could not "dream" the Little Street itself can now digest the published alpha-work of someone who could digest it. [69]

But what happens when such picturing fails? The next month he wrote to Francesca from their home in Croydon to "The Little Cottage" they had just bought in Trimingham, Norfolk.

> I rather felt I wanted to get down to a piece of writing to-day. The worst of it is that there were a number of ideas which had clicked into position and I wished I had managed to get them down, but I didn't. As it is, beyond knowing it was to do with "alpha", I can't remember what they were. And I don't think they always come back. I find it a bit

---

63 16 October 1959, ibid. p. 94.

64 30 October 1959, ibid. p. 102.

65 Undated, ibid. p. 120.

66 14 February 1960, ibid. p. 132.

67 17 February 1960, ibid. p. 133.

68 22 February 1960, ibid. p. 139.

69 24 February, ibid. pp. 143–4.

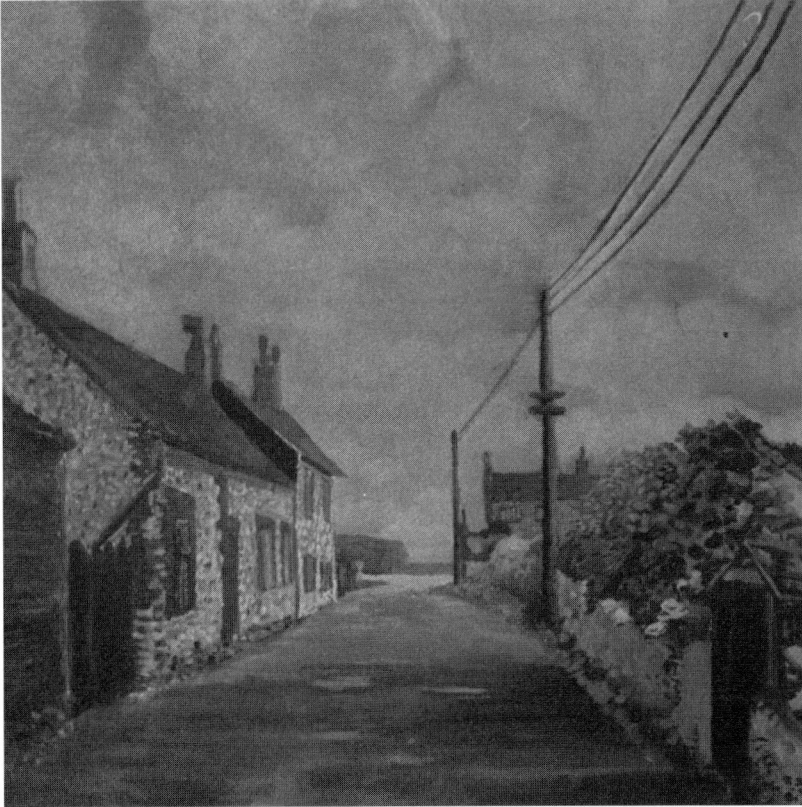

Fig. 11.2 The Little Cottage.

difficult to visualize what you are doing as of course one very cursory look at the cottage is all I have to go by and at present I cannot see it as anything to do with me.[70]

Later he could picture "The Little Cottage". He made a painting of it. (Fig. 11.2). [71] Meanwhile, in unpublished notes, he observed how we sometimes first picture or dream emotional experience when we are asleep because we cannot "permit" ourselves to dream it "during conscious waking life".[72] Either way dreaming renders sense impressions into what Bion called "alpha elements". He said they correspond to what Kant called "phenomena". If they remain unassimilated they are felt, said Bion, to be what Kant called "things-in-themselves". Bion called them

[70] To Francesca, 27 March 1960, Bion 1985 p. 134.

[71] In Bion 1985.

[72] Undated, Bion 1992 p. 150.

"beta elements",[73] just as William James described "the B-region" as "abode of everything that is latent", the source of our "intuitions" and "dreams" (see p. 28 above).[74] To illustrate what he meant by the transformation, and non-transformation of beta into alpha elements, Bion wrote:

> Suppose I am talking to a friend who asks me where I propose to spend my holiday; as he does so, I visualize the church of a small town [Cromer] not far from the village in which I propose to stay. The small town is important because it possesses the railway station nearest to my village. . . . The impressions of the event are being re-shaped as a visual image of that particular church, and so are being made into a form suitable for storage in my mind. By contrast, the patient might have the same experience, the same sense impressions, and yet be unable to transform the experience so that he can store it mentally. But instead, the experience (and his sense impressions of it) remains a foreign body; it is felt as a "thing" lacking any of the quality we usually attribute to thought or its verbal expression.[75]

Bion spoke more about this in a talk in Edinburgh in 1961. Just as he had written in his unpublished notes about the analyst dreaming the emotional experience occurring between him and the patient so as to make it available for learning from experience, he now talked of the mother's "capacity for reverie" as "the receptor organ for the infant's harvest of self-sensation".[76] Her dreaming the baby's feelings turns them, he said, into alpha-elements, into the stuff of conscious and unconscious awareness, attention, and thinking.

Bion's account of this was published in 1962, as was his book, *Learning from Experience*. Whereas Freud implied the existence of a rather rigid boundary repressing unconscious from conscious experience, Bion described a "contact-barrier" allowing selective interchange between them.[77] He contrasted this with psychosis in which, he said, a "beta-element screen" is constructed through projecting everything that could otherwise be dreamt into alpha-elements.[78] He compared this with the baby's early experience. He called the feelings the baby projects "the contained" and the mother into whom they are projected "the container". He represented the resulting link – contained–container – in terms of the male and female symbols for sex, thus evoking the image of the woman taking in the man's penis in making love.

To represent the ineffable – beyond things and words – psychological coupling of patient and analyst in therapy, without using terms already saturated

73 Undated, Bion 1992 p. 157.

74 W. James (1902) *The Varieties of Religious Experience*, London: Fontana, 1960 p. 462.

75 Undated Bion 1992 p. 180.

76 W. R. Bion (1962) A theory of thinking, *IJPA*, **43** pp. 306–310, in Bion 1967 pp. 110–9 16.

77 W. R. Bion (1962) *Learning from Experience*, London: Heinemann, p. 17.

78 Ibid. p. 25.

with pre-assigned meaning, Bion designated the processes involved algebraically. He used the letters L, H, and K to stand for the linking of one person with another in loving, hating, and knowing them. He also devised a grid to represent the development of this linking process in psychoanalysis. He represented, on a vertical axis, progress from raw sense data (beta-elements), through dream-work data (alpha-elements), myths (the social counterpart of dreams), and preconceptions. When mated with their realization, he said, preconceptions become concepts. They in turn become preconceptions for further mating realization, concepts, scientific deduction, and algebraic abstraction. On the horizontal axis of his grid Bion represented the analyst's thinking, beginning with a definitory hypothesis. He warned analysts against prematurely turning this into an interpretation for fear of not knowing. If all goes well, however, when the analyst's initial definitory hypothesis is ready to become saturated with meaning, it progresses to what Bion called "notation" and from this to "attention", "inquiry" and "action".

Attention is also involved, he maintained, in the analyst's preconceptions. He likened the analyst's attention to the patient to the mother attending to what is going on in her baby. This includes, he said, taking in the baby's bad feelings, and transforming them "into feelings of love" such that, in feeding, "the infant sucks its bad property, now translated into goodness, back again".[79] But, unlike mothering, Bion insisted, psychoanalysis involves neither loving nor hating. It involves knowing through putting together the disparate phenomena of the psychoanalytic session to make them whole.

Bion's account of this process was published in 1963. Writing a couple of years later from Norfolk to Francesca, then involved in organizing a consulting room for him in their new home, in Wells Rise, near Primrose Hill, Bion pictured to her "a wonderful sunset – just pure glow of colour, not anything spectacular in the way of clouds – simply radiance. I send it to you with my love. My darling I think of you always."[80] He also pictured to her himself and the children "icy swim . . . gammon lunch with peas (free) and lettuce . . . [rain] drumming on the roof and down the gutters . . . sun . . . splashed paint about, got on with reading".[81]

He continued to liken psychoanalysis to painting – to a painting by Monet, for instance, of "a path through a field sown with poppies".[82] But, whereas the

---

[79] W. R. Bion (1963) *Elements of Psycho-Analysis*, London: Heinemann, p. 31.

[80] To Francesca, 31 December 1964, in Bion 1985 p. 136.

[81] To Francesca, 2 August 1965, ibid. p. 139.

[82] W. R. Bion (1965) *Transformations*, London: Heinemann, p. 1.

painter can see what he paints, Bion noted, the psychoanalyst cannot see the psychological data he portrays in his interpretations.

Transforming O

Perhaps thinking of the invisibility and sensory nothingness of what goes on psychologically between patient and analyst, Bion called its origin "O". O can neither be seen nor known. The analyst's task therefore, said Bion, is to transform O into an experience that can be known. It entails tolerating the frustration of bearing with what cannot be seen or physically sensed. Emphasizing O's nothingness, Bion called it a "no-thing".[83] Its very nothingness and absence, however, he argued, provide space for thinking, for receiving what he called "a thought in search of a meaning".[84] He depicted the emptiness as a female element awaiting a male element to contain.

But the frustration of existence and of the nothingness involved can be so terrifying (as Tillich observed – see p. 126), it may be made into a thing. It may be projected as such "into an 'existing' object in order to eject the 'existing-ness'".[85] One may even seem to see what one projects. Bion gave the example of patients describing what they hallucinatorily see as "penis black with rage" or "eye green with envy".[86] In doing so, he said, the patient makes something out of nothing – out of what Bion called the "noughtness" of O.[87] He likened O to what Plato called the Form of the Good. He described our coming to know it as an instance of what he called a "preconception" and Klein called an "internal object".[88]

It was with this that he brought psychoanalysis together with religion. He likened O to what religious writers have described as "Godhead", "ultimate reality", or "truth".[89] He noted that one religious writer defined Godhead as "spiritual substance, so elemental that we can say nothing about it".[90] In Christian Platonism, Bion went on, O is incarnated in God. Incarnated or not, O itself cannot be known. At best we can be or become O. The analyst's job,

---

[83] W. R. Bion (1965) *Transformations*, London: Heinemann, p. 106.

[84] Ibid. p. 109.

[85] Ibid. p. 112.

[86] Ibid. pp. 114–15.

[87] Ibid. p. 134.

[88] Ibid. p. 138.

[89] Ibid. pp. 139–40.

[90] Ibid. p. 139.

Bion argued, is to enable the patient, through his interpretations, to move from knowing about himself to consenting to become himself – O – of which the supreme example is the mystic experiencing ultimate reality, "won", in Milton's terms, "from the void and formless infinite".[91]

Becoming one with the infinite – with the spirit of life that is eternal yet also unique and limited within each of us—entails embracing the freedom, and "being responsible", [92] that goes with the life of the spirit, rather than reifying or deifying it as a thing or god in oneself or others. Perhaps that is why being or becoming O evokes fear of what Bion called "psychological turbulence".[93] It was this fear, said Bion, that St John of the Cross described in writing:

> The first (night of the soul) has to do with the point from which the soul goes forth, for it has gradually to deprive itself of desire for all the worldly things which it pos-sessed, by denying them to itself; the which denial and deprivation are, as it were, night to all the senses of man. The second reason has to do with the mean, or the road along which the soul must travel to this union – that is, faith, which is likewise as dark as night to the understanding. The third has to do with the point to which it travels – namely, God, Who, equally, is dark night to the soul in this life.[94]

This threefold character of the dark night of the soul, explained Bion, is due to being or becoming O – the ultimate reality of the spirit – entailing first retreat from material reality, second faith in belief rather than knowledge, and third fear lest becoming responsible for oneself make one into a thing-like god. Bion noted that, like St John of the Cross, the mystic, Meister Eckhart, also described emergence from the formlessness of O in threefold terms as only beginning to be knowable in terms of the Trinity—Father, Son, and Holy Ghost.

Just as the mystic is confronted with "the void and formless infinite", wrote Bion, so too are the analyst and patient at the beginning of each session. We might be frightened of this formlessness, like Pascal observing "Le silence éternel de ces éspaces infinis m'effraie".[95] Nevertheless the analyst has to bear with the silence to arrive at a psychologically valid interpretation. In notes for a paper he gave in California a couple of years later, Bion pictured the analyst scrutinizing the session as though it were "elements in a kaleidoscope before they shake into a definable pattern".[96] Bearing with the fragments and their

---

[91] Ibid. p. 151.

[92] Ibid. p. 155.

[93] Ibid. p. 158.

[94] Ibid. pp. 158–9.

[95] Ibid. p. 171.

[96] March 1967, in Bion 1992 p. 290.

integration, and with the persecutory and depressive anxieties this evokes, said Bion, drawing on Klein's theory of paranoid–schizoid and depressive position integration, is nevertheless essential if the borderline or psychotic patient is to accept the analyst's interpretation.[97]

Bion said much the same in summarizing his essays about psychosis. As before he described what he now called the "evolution" of a psychoanalytic session as "the sudden coming together, by a sudden precipitating intuition, of a mass of apparently unrelated incoherent phenomena which are thereby given coherence and meaning not previously possessed".[98] This sudden coming together, he said, depends on intuition. It depends on what Freud, writing about dreams, called consciousness and defined as "the sense-organ for the perception of psychical qualities".[99]

But consciousness of the present is narrowed by memory of what is past and desire for what is to come. Both should therefore be suspended in psychoanalysis. Otherwise, Bion explained, the analyst might be distracted from O as others are by the graven images, idols, and religious statues of what Bion's follower, Neville Symington, calls "primitive religion". [100] In advocating the suspension of memory and desire Bion advocated the same self-emptying as advocated by mystics. Thomas Merton called it "wrestling with blind nought",[101] adding:

> one must learn to act by not acting and to know by not knowing: to have one desire alone which is not really a desire but a kind of desirelessness, an openness, a habitual freedom in the sense of self-abandonment, a realization that all God asks is "that you must turn your attention to Him, and then let Him alone."[102]

Bion also likened psychoanalysis to religion in arguing that neither should aim at cure. For cure, he said, concerns the senses, whereas psychoanalysis and religion are concerned with the psyche or spirit. Criticizing the Gospels for preaching cure – with their tales of Jesus' miracles of healing – Bion argued that this involves the false nostrum "There is a pain. It should be removed. Someone must remove it forthwith, preferably by magic or omnipotence or omniscience, and at once; failing that by science."[103]

....

97 March 1967, in Bion 1992 p. 291.

98 Bion 1967 p. 127.

99 S. Freud (1900) *The Interpretation of Dreams*, **SE5** p. 615, see also Bion 1967 p. 142.

100 N. Symington (1994) *Emotion and Spirit*, London: Cassell, 1998.

101 T. Merton (1961) *Mystics and Zen Masters*, New York: Dell, p. 139.

102 Ibid. p. 138.

103 Bion 1967 p. 149.

But such avoidance of pain obstructs the full attention to reality and truth sought by religion and psychoanalysis. Their churches and institutes ignore this at their peril. Full attention entails becoming aware of what might be new and unfamiliar. This may well be painful and it is never absolute.

Like dreaming when we are asleep, wide-awake attention is never absolutely present nor totally absent. It includes what Jung called "active imagination". Bion described it as the experience in which "some idea or pictorial impression floats into the mind unbidden and as a whole".[104] His daughter, Parthenope, who became a psychoanalyst, linked his account of wide attention, or "psycho-analytic reverie", with what she called "religious contemplation". She said they both might arise out of "a fundamental human necessity",[105] but that since they risk persecutory fear of fragmentation they can perhaps best be tolerated in a state of love.

Simone Weil wrote similarly about love and attention in her book, *Attente de Dieu*, after which it seems possible that Bion's patient, Samuel Beckett, called his play, originally published in French, *En attendant Godot*. Bion was more wary of talking or writing publicly about love. He compared the oneness of attention to whatever emerges to what Keats described in a letter to his brothers as "negative capability" and defined as occurring "when a man is capable of being in uncertainties, mysteries, doubts, without any irritable reaching after fact and reason".[106] At the end of 1967 Bion wrote to Francesca, then looking for a house for them in Los Angeles so that they could get away from the church-like atmosphere of the "Klein Group".[107] He told her about a talk he had given about negative capability. It is a matter of patience. But he was far from patient in waiting for Francesca to be back home with him: "I dare not count the hours and cannot keep from doing it . . . I don't think I can have been in love before. Believe me it's *awful* and lovely at the same time".[108]

At the beginning of 1968 they moved to Brentwood, inland from Santa Monica. Here he wrote of negative capability as a state of mind needed by "thoughts awaiting someone or something to think them".[109] It can give rise to "religious awe", he said, so "incandescent", that some may search – consciously

[104] W. R. Bion (1967) Notes on memory and desire, in E. Bott-Spillius (ed.) *Melanie Klein Today, Volume 2*, London: Routledge, 1988, pp. 17–21, 19.

[105] Bion Talamo p. 54.

[106] In W. R. Bion (1970) *Attention and Interpretation*, London: Heinemann, p. 125.

[107] To Francesca, 3 October 1967, in Bion 1985 p. 146.

[108] To Francesca, 18 October 1967, ibid. p. 149.

[109] Undated – 1969, Bion 1992 p. 304.

or unconsciously – to locate its source in God, the universe, or in another human being.[110]

But he deplored any such false incarnation. He deplored the seduction of evading attention to immediate experience by imagining others or oneself as a hero, genius, or god. He deplored his followers' "Bion – Bion – Bion" accolades.[111] Analysts, he wrote, must divest themselves of all such seductions and grandiosity. They must empty themselves of all memory of the past, desire for the future, and quest for understanding. They must rest content with "faith that there is an ultimate reality and truth – the unknown, unknowable, 'formless infinite' ".[112] He went on to explain that "The exercises in discarding memory and desire must be seen as preparatory to a state of mind in which O can evolve . . . as a step in the process of at-one-ment (the transformation $O \rightarrow K$)."[113]

All too often, Bion went on, in conveying to ordinary people the mystic's "at-one-ment with the deity",[114] religious, psychoanalytic, and other institutions squeeze the life out of this experience. It happened, for instance, when the Catholic Church pilloried Meister Eckhart for apparently claiming oneness with God, "identity with the deity".[115] Undeterred by the fate befalling mystics, Bion himself became increasingly interested in their experience. He told his son Julian that, like the psychoanalyst, Ronnie Laing, he too would like to go to a Buddhist Monastery.[116] He wrote appreciatively to his daughter, Nicola,[117] about a translation by Gerald Brenan of the mystical poems of Saint John of the Cross.

Flying over Dakota in 1972, Bion wrote to Francesca, "The sun is fully up. My goodness, it's time I saw you. It really seems to have been an age. Well – how are you?".[118] It was his last letter to her. They were never separated again. He continued writing, painting, and doing psychoanalysis. He wrote a novel. In it he dwelt on the turbulence of women's and men's love and intimacy with each other, and on the nightmares of his past including trench warfare, rejection, and his first wife's death in childbirth. He also dwelt on his discoveries about religious experience and psychoanalysis. Some passages are akin to conversations in the plays of

---

[110] Undated – 1969, Bion 1992 p. 305.

[111] To Francesca from Amherst College, 21 August 1969, in Bion 1985 p. 159.

[112] Bion 1970 p. 31.

[113] Ibid. p. 33.

[114] Ibid. p. 112.

[115] Ibid. p. 116.

[116] Undated – 1972, in Bion 1985 p. 211.

[117] Undated – 1973, ibid. p. 215.

[118] To Francesca, 22 July 1972, ibid. p. 164.

Beckett. Other passages are akin to Socratic dialogues. He likened the task of the psychoanalyst to that of the philosopher described by Socrates as that of a midwife helping "the soul or psyche to be born".[119]

He described its birth as dependent, in the first instance, on the analyst's silence. "I do not 'excuse' my silence," a psychoanalyst character in his novel says, "but when I want to hear my patients I have to be silent. I listen too for more than is said".[120] He also quoted approvingly the religious poet Gerard Manley Hopkins: "Elected Silence, sing to me/And beat upon my whorlèd ear".[121]

Although he said he only had "hearsay" knowledge of mysticism,[122] he continued to value it highly. It enables one, he said, to see the mystery of variation in constancy, the wisdom of what Confucius called grinding the "mortar of the mind".[123] He wrote of the attention involved in psychoanalysis as being "wide open to what is going on in the session . . . being in the presence of a mystery".[124] It is ineffable. It cannot be seen even though, in madness, it might seem to be visible. An example was a man who, when Bion indicated he had no idea why he came for treatment, said, "I thought you knew. My difficulty is that I blush terribly. I thought you would have noticed it by this time".[125] Yet there was no blushing to be seen. Far from it. He was extremely pale. Yet his blushing was so painfully real to him he dared not go out or have anyone call or phone lest they see it.

By contrast the analyst should be daring. He should have the courage to choose, as evoked by Yeats' poem about a lover choosing whether to marry:

> For though love has a spider's eye
> . . . and tests a lover
> With cruelties of Choice and Chance;
> And when at last that murder's over
> Maybe the bride-bed brings despair,
> For each an imagined image brings
> And finds a real image there.[126]

"One must dare to be aware,"[127] Bion insisted, as he said painters and writers dare in attending to, and "recording their awareness of some sort of influence,

---

[119] W. R. Bion (1980) *Bion in New York and São Paulo*, Perthshire: Cluny Press, p. 97.

[120] Bion 1991 p. 415.

[121] Ibid. pp. 119, 415.

[122] W. R. Bion (1990) *Brazilian Lectures*, London: Karnac, p. 68.

[123] Ibid. p. 118.

[124] Ibid. pp. 127, 131.

[125] Ibid. p. 135.

[126] W. R. Bion (1975) *Caesura*, in W. R. Bion (1989) *Two Papers*, pp. 36–56, 49.

[127] Bion 1992 p. 366.

stimuli that come from without, the unknown that is so terrifying and stimulates such powerful feelings that they cannot be described in ordinary terms".[128] Leonardo da Vinci dared face the chaos, and pictured it in "drawings of water swirling in turmoil, of hair in disorder".[129] Other artists and scientists likewise dare face chaos and disruption even though it is much easier to evade it by dismissing bearers of disruptive new ideas as geniuses or mad, either way as not like us.

Organized religion also often does this. So too do psychoanalytic clinics and institutes. Yet analysis is concerned precisely with the ills done to women and men by just such evasion of the truth. To highlight the point, Bion cited the example of a 30-year-old patient who kept his curtains drawn and insulated himself as much as possible from the world around him:

> He objected to that universe, and at the beginning of the analysis objected to me sufficiently to bring his Smith and Wesson revolver to the sessions; he laid it ostentatiously by his side so as to have available the means of putting a stop to the interpretations. Luckily, or unluckily, having been an instructor in small arms, I paid a great deal of attention to that Smith and Wesson. It did rather distract me from paying attention to what the patient was saying, and I think the patient was similarly saved from having to pay too much attention to what I was saying.[130]

Much better, however, not to be distracted, and not to seek to be distracted from attending to what is going on. Another example of distraction occurred in Bion's analysis of a patient who, at his first session with Bion, could not speak for stammering. Its noise filled the silence. So did other noises: his deep breathing in and out, his swallowing, his straining to fart. His refusal to talk made Bion impatient. How dare this man keep him waiting for the words he wanted. His "spluttering and farting and sucking away with his lips", wrote Bion, evoked the image of a one-man-band. His various organs – mouth, anus, throat, and lips – wanted to be heard all at once. The patient agreed: "they were trying to settle who was top".[131] Overcoming his irritation, saying what he pictured was going on between them, Bion freed his patient to attend to what was going on. With this he began to talk without stammering, and began to discover about the various aspects of himself that wanted to dominate over Bion and his colleagues at work.

128 Bion 1992 p. 369.

129 W. R. Bion (1976) Emotional turbulence, in W. R. Bion (1994) *Clinical Seminars and Other Works*, London: Karnac, pp. 295–306, 296.

130 W. R. Bion (1976) On a quotation from Freud, ibid. pp. 306–11, 309–10.

131 W. R. Bion (1971) The grid, in Bion 1989 pp. 1–33, 18.

Valuing attention, Bion cited approvingly Freud's commendation of Charcot as like an artist, "a man who sees" (see p. 35).[132] But seeing and attending to what is going on – mystically contemplating it – is not necessarily easy. For reality can be unpleasant and unwelcome. "If we cannot get out of it," Bion noted in his very last paper given in March 1979, "if it is not appropriate to run away or to retire," we might escape by "going to sleep or becoming unconscious".[133] That September he returned with Francesca from California to England. They settled in Oxford with plans, later that year, to visit India, home of the *Bhagavad Gita* and its discussion of faith, doing, and knowing, which he often commended in his work. But in early November he became ill. Anticipating the diagnosis, he told a colleague, "Life is full of surprises, mostly unpleasant".[134] The news was unpleasant. He had myeloid leukaemia and died the same week, on 8 November 1979. In a memorial meeting early the next year Francesca quoted a stanza by the same religious poet, George Herbert, whose poem, *Love*, Simone Weil used to recite. It was a stanza Bion had often recited when he woke:

Sweet day, so cool, so calm, so bright,
The bridall of the earth and skie:
The dew shall weep thy fall to night;
For thou must die.

Bion too is dead. But his ideas about psychoanalysis and religion still flourish.

Bion today: Neville Symington

Particularly helpful in explaining the link Bion made between religion and psychoanalysis is the work of Neville Symington. Educated in a Benedictine school, Ampleforth, after which he became a Catholic priest, Symington now works as a psychoanalyst in Australia. In a book called *Emotion and Spirit*, he wrote about ways of uniting religion with psychoanalysis in terms of the distinction made by Erich Fromm between "primitive" and "mature" religion involving projecting and not projecting the freedom of one's spirit into God. Together with his wife, Joan, Symington has also written usefully about the continuity of Bion's ideas about psychoanalysis and religion: from his early observations of group therapy patients evading proto-mental phenomena occurring in the group through making him into a thing-like god; through his subsequent account of analysts containing, dreaming, and thereby transforming the "beta-element" data of the patient's experience into assimilable "alpha-element"

[132] S. Freud (1893) Charcot, **SE3** pp. 11–23, 12.

[133] W. R. Bion (1979) Making the best of a bad job, in Bion 1994 pp. 321–31, 322.

[134] In J. Sayers (2000) *Kleinians*, Cambridge: Polity, p. 132.

form; to his final likening of this process to the mystic's "at-one-ment" with unknowable "ultimate reality" or "O" as means of transforming it into something that can be known.[135]

But Symington also goes beyond Bion. Although, in bringing psychoanalysis together with religion and mysticism, Bion was arguably inspired by love, Bion said little about love in his writing about psychoanalysis. Symington too is wary about writing or talking about love. But he is not as wary as Bion. Bion, as we have seen, was also wary of memory, desire, and understanding. He thereby risked rendering the religious or contemplative stance he advocated psychoanalysts to adopt in doing psychoanalysis too passive. Symington, by contrast, adopts a more active stance. In this his approach is similar to that of Simone Weil emphasizing the active, outward-looking orientation by love of religious attention. It is also similar to Marion Milner's emphasis on actively wide attention in her experiments with mysticism.

In drawing on Bion's work in bringing together psychoanalysis and religion, Symington also emphasizes attention actively oriented outwardly by love. He likens the psychoanalyst, as does Bion, to a mother who, he says, through her "loving act" of "related-to-the-object" active contemplation of the "actual contours" of her baby finds and brings alive his soul or spirit which is both infinite and unique in him.[136] Symington also describes how, when this loving act is absent, the vacuum may be filled by making a god of oneself or others. The spirit thereby becomes a thing. It becomes meaningless. Reviving the life of the spirit can be painful. For it means shouldering freedom and responsibility for choosing and deciding. The burden, Symington claims, is conveyed in Piero della Francesca's painting of Christ with downcast eyes on being anointed by John the Baptist. Patients in therapy may be similarly downcast.

> When someone comes to the consulting room, there are obviously some embers left that are in hope that something can arise from within and start to put these pieces together again. There is also a tremendous force against it the whole time because whenever things have shattered out of some pain, as they are put together again, the pain is re-experienced.[137]

Many would prefer to remain in what one of his patients called a "tortoiseshell state".[138]

---

[135] J. Symington and N. Symington (1996) *The Clinical Thinking of Wilfred Bion*, London: Routledge.

[136] N. Symington (2001) *The Spirit of Sanity*, London: Karnac, pp. 65, 73.

[137] Ibid. p. 107.

[138] Ibid. pp. 121–2.

Health, however, is not a shell or thing. It is life. A hospitalized alcoholic told Symington his own recovery to health began when, driven by a thing-like impulse to kill himself or smash the hospital window, he suddenly thought, "Or I could decide to get better".[139] How can psychoanalysts enable their patients similarly to take responsibility for deciding and choosing? To revive their patients' spirit, their "conscience", says Symington, analysts must engage in the same act of loving contemplation as mystics and mothers. And this depends, he claims, on the analyst having had enough analysis to be able to know and face his own fears in "surrender to a good, loving principle".[140] It entails, says Symington, an "act of faith" like the mystic seeking, through contemplation, to purify the spirit of its false gods – "its anthropomorphic accretions".[141]

A clinical example, Symington maintains, was a woman patient who, coming into analysis after a very bad breakdown, initially only referred to things in his room – "clock", "book", and so on. Using his imagination, Symington put the pieces together as best he could. Perhaps it enabled her to dream, or at least to remember her dreams. After a while she told him one. She had dreamt, she said, of the body of her mother, which, when she went over to touch it, blew into a thousand pieces. Paradoxically, through being integrated into a dream, arguably helped by being previously integrated through Symington's imagination and interpretations, the fragments of her experience came together. She began to get better. But although Symington mentions love in such contexts, he is guarded about it. Perhaps it is not surprising that it is women, more than men, who have emphasized love in relation to psychoanalysis and religion: including Bion's psychoanalyst daughter, Parthenope, as mentioned above; and, particularly influentially, Julia Kristeva, whom interestingly Symington criticizes on this account. Essentially, he argues, whilst English-speaking analysts focus on truth, Kristeva "places love as the motivating centre of the analytic exchange".[142] Indeed she does.

[139] Ibid. p. 26.

[140] Ibid. p. 21.

[141] Ibid. p. 161.

[142] N. Symington (1991) Review of *In the Beginning was Love* by Julia Kristeva, *Free Associations*, 2(3), pp. 462–6, 463.

Chapter 12

Julia Kristeva

Mothering holiness

Despite, or perhaps because it is extremely difficult to understand what Julia Kristeva writes, she is much celebrated both in her adopted country France, and by academics across the world for her writing about love, psychoanalysis, and religion. Born in 1941 in Bulgaria into a Russian Orthodox family, she was taught at primary school by French nuns. As a teenager, she says, she was inspired by reading Dostoevsky into seeking to acquire her family's religion. But she found she preferred the immortality of ideas to the immortality of God: "What need, what wish for a supreme being", she asked, "since thought could endure without me?"[1]

So, like her father, Stoian Kristev, who was an eminent scholar, she devoted herself to ideas, to becoming an intellectual. She studied Russian formalism, and in 1965, went to France to study with Roland Barthes in Paris. Here she married the novelist and editor of *Tel Quel*, Philippe Sollers, with whom she has a son, David, born in 1976. The same year she also began training as a psychoanalyst and with her essay "Stabat mater",[2] published that year, began writing increasingly about holiness and mothering and more generally about love, psychoanalysis and religion, as I will illustrate and explain after first recounting other developments at this time in feminism and psychoanalysis with which her work is very much allied.

Feminism and psychoanalysis

The US black civil rights movement, together with protest against the US war in Vietnam, and student movement uprisings in Paris and elsewhere in 1968, were a major impetus for the then revival of feminism in the USA and Europe. Many feminists turned against Freud and the popularization of psychoanalysis,

---

[1] J. Kristeva, 4 February 1997, in C. Clément and J. Kristeva (1998) *Le féminin et le sacré*, Paris: Stock, p. 78.

[2] J. Kristeva (1976) *Stabat mater*, in J. Kristeva (1983) *Tales of Love*, New York: Columbia University Press, pp. 234–63.

particularly within US psychiatry, and its repudiation of feminism as the effect of neurotic penis envy.[3] In England feminists also turned against Melanie Klein, Winnicott, and other psychoanalysts – particularly John Bowlby – for the use made of their emphasis on the importance of early mothering for the baby's subsequent mental health as a reason for closing publicly funded day nurseries opened during the war to enable mothers to work.[4] Feminists have also criticized psychoanalysts, particularly Winnicott, for idealizing mothering thereby leading to unwarranted mother-blaming when things go wrong.[5] Subsequently, however, feminists have also used Winnicott's account of the oneness of mothers with their baby daughters, as well as with their baby sons, to explain the reproduction of social inequalities between the sexes.[6] Feminist therapists have also used the mother-centred work of Winnicott and other psychoanalysts in seeking to understand and treat the ills done women and men by sexual inequality.[7]

Others, by contrast, have adopted the work of the Paris-based psychoanalyst, Jacques Lacan.[8] Taking issue with those, like Erich Fromm, who centre psychoanalysis on the individual self or ego, Lacan argued that the assumption that the ego is essentially healthy and whole is an illusion based on the baby's imagined oneness with his unified image of himself in the mirror when, in reality, he is fragmented by the cross-cutting drives of the id. Divided between these two senses of himself – as fragmented and whole – the toddler, said Lacan, subsequently entertains a further illusion, namely that of being one with what his mother most desires. But this illusion too is shattered.

Through the castration complex, as described by Freud, Lacan argued, the child discovers the presence of a penis in boys but not in girls, and thereby discovers the meaning of the phallus which, said Lacan, is given by this antithesis. The child thereby discovers that the phallus symbolizes love and sex, and is indeed a central symbol in patriarchal society. Furthermore, Lacan claimed, the child learns through the Oedipus complex the law of the father prohibiting him from being or having the phallus the mother desires.

....

[3] e.g. B. Friedan (1963) *The Feminine Mystique*, Harmondsworth: Penguin, 1965; K. Millett (1971) *Sexual Politics*, New York: Avon Books.

[4] e.g. D. Riley (1983) *War in the Nursery*, London: Virago.

[5] e.g. J. Doane and D. Hodges (1992) *From Klein to Kristeva*, Ann Arbor: University of Michigan Press.

[6] e.g. N. Chodorow (1978) *The Reproduction of Mothering*, Berkeley: University of California Press.

[7] e.g. S. Orbach (1978) *Fat is a Feminist Issue*, New York: Paddington Press.

[8] See e.g. E. Grosz (1990) *Jacques Lacan: A Feminist Introduction*, London: Routledge.

In sum, the child's subjectivity is formed, according to Lacan, by the prevailing symbolic order of our society represented, within Christianity, by the word of God. Freud represented this state of affairs in terms of the psyche being constituted by three agencies – the id, ego, and superego. Lacan theorized them as mediating respectively "the Real", "the Imaginary", and "the Symbolic". They involve, respectively, the reality of the child's biological instincts or drives, the imaginary oneness of the child with his mirror image, and the child's initiation into the meaning of the phallus and law of the father through the castration and Oedipus complex.

The semiotic

Some feminists, Julia Kristeva among them, argue that Lacan's theory provides a means of understanding how men and women come to be positioned as subject or object in patriarchal social relations, in terms of having or being the phallus. Kristeva also goes beyond Lacan. She emphasizes the precursors of symbolism in what Winnicott described as the baby's use of sounds and words of the adults around him in creating and naming his first not-me possession or transitional object (see p. 192). Kristeva calls this first form of language "semiotic".

She links it with religion. In doing so she draws attention, like many others, to the decline of religion in nineteenth century Europe and thereby means of giving life and shape to the psyche or spirit through religious rites, rituals, and sacraments. In literature, she says, the resulting void has been filled by modernist writers such as Mallarmé, Joyce, Proust, Artaud, and Céline. To this one could add that Jung and Freud also filled the void by encouraging their patients to express and give life and form to the individuality of their soul or psyche, not in standard terms authorized by Christian or Jewish religion, but in terms of the individually unique free associations, active imagination, fantasies and dreams, they encouraged their patients to draw and tell.

Kristeva's originality lies in her adding that mothers have in effect always done this. They have always encouraged and thereby brought into being the holiness, as it were, of their babies' soul or spirit through their oneness with their babies. In this, emphasizes Kristeva, mothers are also aware of their separateness from their babies in relating to someone or something else – to the baby's father, for instance, or to their work. Imagining herself into her baby's shoes, as Winnicott put it, the mother, says Kristeva, animates her baby's psyche or soul through articulating his bodily drives – hunger, thirst, sex, and so on – by transforming them into the distinctive marks, traces, precursory signs, imprints, figures, rhythms, music, sounds, hesitations, pauses, silences and so on that she equates with the underlying semiotic texture of language.

Psychoanalysts, she argues, likewise bring the life of their patients' soul or psyche into being through loving oneness with them. In this, she says, they follow Christ's commandment: "Thou shalt love thy neighbour as thyself".[9] Through empathic love of their patients psychoanalysts are able to bring their patients' soul to life through giving it semiotic as well as symbolic shape and form. To illustrate this I will recount separately how Kristeva describes this as happening in psychoanalytic treatment of phobia and psychosis, melancholia, "the sick soul", guilt and anorexia, and in the mothering of child analysis.

Phobia and psychosis

Bion argues, in effect, that through his at-one-ment with the unmediated ultimate reality (which Lacan calls the Real) of what goes on psychologically in the patient, and between the patient and himself, the analyst contains, dreams, and thereby transforms and mediates it into a form that can be registered and known, consciously or unconsciously, by the patient. Bion argues that mothers ideally do the same with their babies. He also argues that, if the mother is unable to fulfil this mediating, transforming function, or if the baby is too envious of this function in the mother, then it may experience its re-internalized, previously projected, self-sensations, as "nameless dread".[10] Or, if it cannot bear frustration, it may experience the absence of the mother's breast, for instance, not as the beginning of a thought such as "no-breast", but as a thing, as a "bad object" to be got rid of. Bion explains in these terms what has been called the thought disorder and concrete thinking of psychosis, phobias, and obsessions.

Kristeva likewise explains religion. Whereas, in his book *Totem and Taboo*, Freud explained the ritual practices of religion as originating in atonement for patriarchal murder, Kristeva explains religious rituals in feminist terms as means of warding of male-dominated society's horror of what is female and feminine, and equated with nature. Specifically she describes mysogynist dread of becoming submerged in, and one with one's mother as one was in the womb. With the decline of religion, says Kristeva, psychoanalysis has emerged as a means of treating phobic and psychotic exclusion of such terrors from

----

[9] Gospel according to St Matthew ch. 22 verse 39.

[10] W. R. Bion (1962) A theory of thinking, in W. R. Bion (1967) *Second Thoughts*, London: Heinemann, pp. 110–20, 116.

thinking and speaking. Through empathic love of and oneness with the patient, the analyst is able to give what otherwise surfaces in nameless dread, free-floating anxiety, or in rigid phobic or psychotic defences, means of expressing, thinking about and thereby allaying the nameless or formless source of dread and anxiety through giving it semiotic and symbolic form and shape.

The phobic patient, in effect, says to the analyst, argues Kristeva, "I displace, therefore your must associate and condense for me". In short, she goes on, "[He] is asking the analyst to build up an imagination for him. He is asking to be saved like Moses, to be born like Christ. He is asking for a rebirth".[11] Kristeva interprets in these terms Freud's successful treatment of a 4-year-old boy, Little Hans, through enabling his father to put into words Hans' horror of being castrated, agoraphobically displaced onto fear of horses biting him in the street.

To illustrate her claim that it is through loving identification with the patient that, like the Winnicottian "good enough" mother, the psychoanalyst resurrects the patient's love and spirit, Kristeva describes the case of a border-line psychotic patient, John. She describes how, in analysis with her, John talked of incest and murder as though they were meaningless things. Narcissistically obsessed with himself, he was unconscious of any love for others, until this was evoked and revived, according to Kristeva, through his transference-love for her. With this he began to be able to give his feelings shape. They included feelings of revulsion as well as of love. He described himself, as well as his mother, as repulsive: his motto – "I am repulsive, there-fore I am". Dreams also emerged, including one of protecting himself from his mother's lover by running away, and only being saved by an old man miracul-ously appearing, St Christopher, "the one who carries Jesus . . . He carries me, but my own feet are doing the walking".[12]

This perhaps contributed to John, in subsequent sessions, beginning to remember again his mother's brother and her father with whom he had spent his early years. He also remembered his own father. Previously he had dispar-aged and dismissed him. Now he spoke warmly of him as an "unassuming intellectual", "movie buff", "reader of James".[13] In evoking his love and becom-ing one not so much with his mother but with his father, it seems, Kristeva enabled John to give shape to what was otherwise a source of nameless dread

---

[11] J. Kristeva (1980) *Powers of Horror*, New York: Columbia University Press, 1982, p. 50.

[12] J. Kristeva (1983) *Tales of Love*, New York: Columbia University Press, 1998, p. 49.

[13] Ibid. p. 50.

and horror, equated by Kristeva with what she calls the abjection of being reincorporated into nature and the mother's womb.

Melancholia

Another example of abjection, says Kristeva, is melancholia. Freud described it as resulting from defending against disillusion, separation, and loss through identifying with those we love as though they were the same as us. Criticizing this defensive illusion, Kristeva approvingly cites Plato's observations regarding our yearning to become one with another – as embodiment of the Form of the Good – represented by Psyche, led by Eros, becoming one with the divine. Kristeva also repeats Plato's homily, in *The Symposium*, that separation is the precondition of love, of wanting someone out there, other than us, that we do not have. Separation is also the condition of the psyche or soul coming into being. Love, says Kristeva, enables the soul to emerge from nothingness. For the essence of love resides in its other-directedness with which, in mysticism, she says, subject and object become one. Or, as Kristeva also puts it, "The love of God and for God resides in a gap: the broken space made explicit by sin on the one side, the beyond on the other".[14]

Combining St John's assertion, "God is love", with the first sentence of St John's gospel, "In the beginning was the Word, and the Word was with God, and the Word was God", Kristeva argues in another book, *In the Beginning was Love*, that people seek psychoanalysis because they lack love. In evoking their love, in giving it semiotic and symbolic shape and form, psychoanalysts, she says, like Christianity, restore to their patients their ability to love and to know about their love.

An alternative is the oneness of mysticism. Countering the father-centredness of Freudian psychoanalysis with the mother-centredness of Winnicottian and Bionian feminist psychoanalysis, Kristeva describes recovery of fusion with another on a "semiotic" and maternal rather than "symbolic" and paternal and phallocentric basis. In doing so she quotes in her support St Augustine likening Christian faith in God to the baby at the breast. Psychoanalysts, she says, similarly begin with faith in just such loving oneness of one with another, of the baby with the mother, of the analysand with the analyst.

Freud never doubted the illusory character of this oneness with others in being in love. But, claims Kristeva, Freud also recognized how much we need such illusions. Actually, as we have seen, this is not true of Freud. More accurately Kristeva notes that Freud's followers emphasize our need of illusion – specifically the illusion of oneness with another – as a means to psychological

---

[14] Ibid. pp. 161–2.

creativity and mental health. Psychoanalysis, she says, in keeping with her post-modern deconstructionist philosophy, seeks to preserve us from certainty. Hence its enthusiasm for illusion and mysticism. Unlike mysticism, however, psychoanalysis, she says, not only seeks to enable patients to recover oneness with another but also to dissolve this oneness so as to enable them to recognize themselves as separate and different from the analyst as the analyst is from them.

This returns me to melancholia. Freud, as I have said before, described melancholia as a condition in which, defending against separation from, and disappointment in those we love, we imagine ourselves to be one with them. They thereby become an ideal and judgemental figure within us. Hence, said Freud, the self-complaints of the depressed housewife complaining against herself that she is worthless and no good. Fused and identified with another, adds Kristeva, the melancholic is deprived of the space between herself or himself and others that is the precondition of love. The melancholic, says Kristeva, is akin to the mystic imprisoned in "ineffable" feeling beyond words. Religious language, she says, provides a semiotic and symbolic means of struggling against this collapse of feeling in melancholic fusion of oneness with another. Creative writing can do the same. So too, says Kristeva, can psychoanalysis.

As an example she describes the case of a depressed patient, Anne, who had lost all enthusiasm for life. She broke up what little she said with silence, making her speech unintelligible. Empathically imagining herself into Anne's plight, Kristeva talked to her about her uneasiness whenever she came close, in words, to her sadness. Knowing also that Anne had suffered with various skin diseases as a baby, Kristeva put this too into words. She talked about this experience with Anne in terms of her retreating into her skin as a baby faced with her mother's seeming or actual resistance to holding or touching her then. Through these and other interpretations, it seems, Kristeva opened up a space between Anne and the illusory fusion of her melancholia with her mother, and between Anne and her illusory fusion with Kristeva. It resulted, Kristeva indicates, in Anne being able to give her feelings – hate as well as love – form in the shape of dreams and words. She recounted, for instance, the following dream on returning from holiday: "There was a trial, like [Klaus] Barbie's trial: I handled the prosecution, everyone was convinced. Barbie was found guilty".[15] In her dream Anne felt relieved as if she had been freed from a torturer. But she was not there. She was somewhere else. She felt hollow. She preferred not

---

[15] J. Kristeva (1987) *Black Sun*, New York: Columbia University Press, 1989, p. 57.

to wake up. She wanted to stay asleep. Imagining herself into Anne's dream, and thinking about her complaining of feeling empty, hollow, and sterile, Kristeva commented:

> On the surface there are torturers [*tortionnaires*]. Further away, however, or elsewhere, where your sorrow lies, there is perhaps: *Torse-io-naître/pas naître* [torsion between being and not being born].[16]

At this Anne talked of her fear of never giving birth. Kristeva's interpretation, it seems, also enabled her to imagine, dream, and put this fear into words:

> I dreamt that a little girl came out of my body. She was the spitting image of my mother whose face, when I close my eyes, as I have often told you, I cannot bring to mind, as if she had died before I was born and carried me along with her into death. And now here I am giving birth and it is her who lives again.[17]

In thus dreaming and telling her dream she gave expression to an achievement of her analysis. Arguably this achievement was won through Kristeva's imaginative oneness with Anne enabling her to interpret and put into words Anne's otherwise silent misery. Writers and artists likewise give shape to what otherwise remains a silent, unpictured, unverbalised source of melancholic fusion and sadness. Examples, says Kristeva, include Holbein's painting, *The Body of the Dead Christ in The Tomb*, and Dostoevsky's account of it in his novel, *The Idiot*.

The sick soul

In *The Varieties of Religious Experience* William James depicts what he calls "the sick soul" as an alienated divided self reborn and transformed into wholeness and health through oneness with God. In her book, *New Maladies of the Soul*, Kristeva likewise describes the sickness of the soul. She attributes its increasing prevalence to people becoming alienated from their psyche or spirit through adopting the hand-me-down, quick-fix imagery of today's mass media society.

To illustrate the transforming rebirth of the soul from sickness into health through psychoanalysis, Kristeva recounts the case of an artist, Didier. He arrived in analysis, she says, complaining of loneliness, inability to love, and of indifference to his wife, colleagues and to the death of his mother. He was only interested in painting and masturbating. He was not bothered by his mother dying, except that she was the only person whom he had allowed to see his paintings.

---

[16] Ibid. p. 58.

[17] Ibid. p. 58.

In analysis with Kristeva he only began to come to life in talking with her about his paintings. His soul was also arguably further enlivened by Kristeva putting into words the images the violence of his paintings and collages of cut-up posters, drenched or daubed with colour, evoked in her. In accepting, changing, and rejecting her understanding of his pictures, he named the fantasies they expressed. His fantasies came to replace his previous unthinking acting out his feelings in violence and masturbation. In naming and giving words to his feelings in the form of fantasy he was also enabled to give them form in the shape of dreams. They included dreams about his father. In telling them Didier was also able to recover in words the disappointment and anger he felt at his father for not intervening to stop his mother dominating over him as a child, treating him as her passive pawn, and dressing him up as a girl. When his treatment ended he gave Kristeva a picture he had painted of her. Kristeva comments: "By painting my portrait and accompanying it with his own commentary, Didier gave me what I had given him . . . the 'logos of the soul'".[18]

Guilt

The soul or psyche, of course, are central to both religion and psychoanalysis. Both are also concerned, Kristeva emphasizes, with guilt and with the remission, redemption, and forgiveness of sins, as in the Christian prayer to God: "Forgive us our trespasses as we forgive them who trespass against us". But one can only be forgiven in so far as one is conscious of having done wrong. Repressing or projecting knowledge of, and guilt about our wrongdoing into an internal superego or external judge makes wrongdoing unconscious. Repression or projection makes it into an alien and meaningless thing. As such guilt is a major cause of psychiatric disorder – of neurotic anxiety, panic, depression, auditory hallucinations, and so on.

Its treatment in psychoanalysis entails becoming conscious of guilt not as a thing but as the effect of an intended wrongdoing. Discovering the underlying, unconscious intention, suggests Kristeva, depends on analysts identifying with this intention in their patients through oneness with them in knowing about the intentions in their own wrongdoing. The patient's wrongdoing also becomes evident in the patient's and analyst's transference relation with each other. Without discovering the unconscious intention lying behind the

---

[18] J. Kristeva (1993) *New Maladies of the Soul*, New York: Columbia University Press, 1995, p. 26.

patient's wrongdoing it remains meaningless, a thing, outside the sphere of what can be forgiven.

Forgiveness is only possible once the patient becomes conscious of the intention motivating his wrongdoing. It does not absolve it, but it does entail bringing about the rebirth of the patient's spirit in choosing and being responsible for choosing whether to do right or wrong. Or as Kristeva also puts it (at least as I understand her):

> Forgiveness – that is to say, the gift of meaning at the heart of the transference – is also at the heart of the talking cure of psychoanalysis. Not that forgiveness through psychoanalysis absolves wrongdoing. From beneath action, it involves the encounter of the patient's unconscious with a loving other, who does not judge, but who understands the patient's truth without acting on the love that enables their rebirth.[19]

Another way of understanding all this is in terms of the story told by Dostoevsky in his novel, *Crime and Punishment*. It tells the tale of a student, Raskolnikov, tormented with anxiety and panic after butchering to death an old woman money-lender. Convinced of his rightness in killing her, he only becomes reborn – resurrected, as Dostoevsky puts it – through love of a woman, Sonya, enabling him to become aware, if only glimmeringly, of the wrong he has done. Kristeva herself explains this both in terms of Dostoevsky's *Crime and Punishment* and also in terms of anorexia.

Anorexia

Kristeva locates anorexia in a religious context. She tells the story of a seventeenth century saint, Catherine of Sienna, driven seemingly by unconscious guilt about having survived her twin and many of her other siblings, including her slightly younger sister, Giovanna. This unconscious guilt, it seems, drove Catherine consciously to rebel against her mother's order that she marry her dead sister's husband by becoming a nun, and by starving herself to death. Subsequently she was sanctified by the Roman Catholic church because of the miracle of her mystical union, in life, with God. Kristeva, however, indicates that Catherine was neither truly holy nor truly a saint. Not only did she disavow her bodily life through her self-starvation, she also denied the life of

---

[19] "Le par-don – c'est-à-dire *le don de signifiance à l'intérieur du transfert* – serait ainsi l' économie interne de la parole analytique. Vous comprenez que ce par-don-ci ne lave pas les actes. Sous les actes, il lève l'inconscient et lui fait rencontrer un autre, amoureux: un autre qui ne juge pas, mais entend 'ma' vérité dans la disponibilité de l'amour et, pour cela même, permet de renaître". J. Kristeva, 16 January 1996, *Le pardon peut-il guérir?* in J. Kristeva (1997) *La révolte intime*, Paris: Fayard, pp. 23–39, 32.

her spirit through remaining unconscious of the wrongdoing and guilt driving her to starve herself.

Kristeva tells Catherine's story in connection with an anorexic patient, Agnes. She suggests that Agnes became aware of the unconscious wrongdoing causing her symptoms through Kristeva's loving identification with Agnes reminding her of her own wrongdoing as a baby in rejecting both concentrated and skimmed milk of cows and goats when her mother could not feed her herself because her breasts had become infected. Through thus recalling her own feelings of wrongdoing in oneness with Agnes, it seems, Kristeva enabled her to become conscious of the wrongdoing driving her anorexia and bulimia. In Agnes' case it seemingly involved the fantasy of becoming involved in her parents' love-making and wanting to eat her mother. In becoming conscious of this the severity of Agnes' otherwise alien-seeming, thing-like superego driving her to binge and starve was dissolved. She became more able to talk and write in and through her analysis.

Mothering

Kristeva recounts her psychoanalytic treatment of Agnes' anorexia in a book about femininity and holiness. In it Kristeva dwells on what she calls the serenity of the mother's love for her baby. She describes it as successor to the mother's erotic satisfaction in the baby's father (or work, or whatever). In mothering, she says, a woman's love becomes absorbed in looking after and cultivating someone else. Beyond mothering, she adds, there is nothing else in human experience which so radically involves bringing into being the emergence of another.[20] Kristeva also puts this in religious terms, in terms of Russian Orthodox iconography. Its image of the Virgin Mary, she says, evokes particularly well the serenity of mothering. Communion with her ineffable maternal magic restores oneness with God and, in the process, transforms both us and nature.[21]

Kristeva also puts this in secular terms. She dwells on what she calls the "feminine genius" of women in bringing their babies' psyche and soul into

---

[20] "l' 'object' de satisfaction érotique qu'est le père (ou telle relation, profession, gratification . . .), se résorbe doucement en 'autre' – à soigner, à cultiver . . . . Hors la maternité, il'nexiste pas, dans l'expérience humaine, de situations qui nous confrontent aussi radicalement et aussi simplement à cette émergence de l'autre". Kristeva, 17 March 1997, in Clément and Kristeva p. 93.

[21] "La communion avec l'innommable envoûtement maternel . . . permet de restaurer l'union avec la divinité, de transfigurer l'homme et la nature". Kristeva, 18 April 1997, ibid. p. 126.

being. She discusses in these terms the work of Hannah Arendt. Inspired by love of Heidegger, she says, Arendt devoted her thesis to St Augustine's concept of love as entailing love of another not for what they are but for what we want them to become. So too with mothering: "Mother love", says Kristeva, "is perhaps the dawn of our tie with another, which the lover and mystic discover later".[22] It involves love of whatever is new in the other. Through mother love, claims Kristeva, the holiness, which religious man transmutes to everyday life, shines out.[23]

Child analysis

Kristeva also illustrates this in terms of child analysis with examples from the work of Melanie Klein. Kristeva describes Klein, like Arendt, as also a feminine genius in using her unconscious intuition of what went on in her adult and child patients' minds as the means of dreaming into shape their otherwise psychologically meaningless impulses and drives. As illustration Kristeva recounts Klein's account of her analysis of her son, Erich, when he was four. Kristeva describes how, through telling him the story about the woman whose husband wished a sausage would grow on the end of his nose, Klein inspired Erich, who had previously been inhibited from playing and storytelling, into giving his impulses narrative shape and form. It inspired him to tell stories, including a convoluted tale about two cows walking together, one jumping on the other, going to hell, finding the devil, and eventually going to a castle, pricking themselves like Sleeping Beauty, falling asleep, and a hundred years later waking up to be greeted by a king.

Kristeva also illustrates the analyst intuiting and bringing to life her child patient's fantasies with the example of Klein's analysis of her 4-year-old autistic patient, Dick. Kristeva argues that, through imaginatively identifying with Dick, as a mother lovingly identifies with her baby, Klein played out fantasies he might have entertained, of himself for instance, as a train going into his mother as a station (see p. 153). Through projective identification oneness with Dick, says Kristeva, Klein enabled the "ineffable proto-symbolism" of Dick's bodily drives and impulses to come into psychological being.[24] In this Kristeva draws on Bion's notion of at-one-ment with O enabling its transformation into something that can be known. She likens such transformation to the transubstantiation of bread and wine into the body and blood of Christ in

---

[22] J. Kristeva (1999) *Hannah Arendt*, Paris: Fayard, p. 83.

[23] Ibid. p. 85.

[24] J. Kristeva (2000) *Melanie Klein*, Paris: Fayard, p. 260.

Holy Communion, and to the transubstantiation of everyday objects described by Proust as achieved by the painter, Chardin.

> Chardin has taught us that a pear is as living as a woman, a kitchen crock as beautiful as an emerald. He has proclaimed the divine quality of all things under the light which beautifies them and to the mind which reflects on them.[25]

Kristeva suggests that just as Chardin brings to life "the divine quality of all things" in his painting, so too Klein brought to life the spirit in Dick through enacting fantasies he might have had about his mother. Certainly her playing with trains in these terms enabled him to become alive to, or at least conscious of, feelings to which he was previously numb. But there is a danger in mothers and psychoanalysts projectively identifying with what they imagine their children and patients might feel. In doing so they risk freezing and deadening the spirit of those in their care through falsifying the truth of their feelings. Bion sought to protect patients from this risk by emphasizing that psychoanalysts should guard against prematurely saturating their preconceptions, formulations, and interpretations of the raw data of their patients' experience with pre-given theories and meanings. Instead they should keep their interpretations open to further "mating", as he put it, with whatever realizations their at-one-ment with the psychological reality evolving between them and their patients might subsequently reveal.

Kristeva evidently values and adopts many of Bion's insights. But she says little about his thus advocating that psychoanalysts adopt a scientific, hypothesis-testing method in their work. Instead, with her adherence to Lacan's theory of symbolism, and her theory of the semiotic, she risks making her unification of psychoanalysis and religion into rigid structuralist and post-structuralist dogma.

Mystery-making

Possibly Kristeva's overlooking of science is also due to her love of mystery. She acknowledges her nostalgia for her childhood home's orthodox faith – "its sensuality, its mystery, that seclusion that makes us feel, in the celebration of the liturgy, the sorrows and joys of another world".[26] Perhaps her love of mystery also contributes to Kristeva making what she writes so convoluted,

25 M. Proust (c.1909) *By Way of Sainte-Beuve*, London: Chatto & Windus, pp. 249–50. Kristeva writes about these and other insights of Proust in e.g. J. Kristeva (1993) *Proust and the Sense of Time*, London: Faber.

26 J. Kristeva (1995) Bulgaria, my suffering, in J. Kristeva (2000) *Crisis of the European Subject*, New York: Other Press, pp. 165–83, 177.

abstract, and mysterious that it is sometimes impossible, or almost impossible, to understand what she says. This is particularly the case in the book *Tales of Love*, in which she most seeks to bring together love, psychoanalysis, and religion. Nevertheless what I understand, perhaps mistakenly, from what I have read of her writing very much informs what I have said in this book. What, to conclude, has it all been about?

Conclusion

I said at the beginning that this book is a love story. I have sought to tell the tale of how psychotherapy, born of love, is rediscovering love in relation to religion. Another way of conceptualizing this story is in terms of a revolution occurring in psychotherapy from the individualistic stance of William James to the interpersonal, intersubjective stance of Kristeva.

I began with William James' account of people recovering wholeness and health through their experience, as individuals, of oneness with God. I then turned to Freud's development of psychoanalysis as means of enabling people to recover from unconsciousness their individually-given instincts towards love and sex. Next I outlined Jung's theory of health through individuation, through recovering oneness of consciousness with the unconscious. Simone Weil too regarded recovery from affliction as an individual matter of willing oneself to turn one's attention to God. Erich Fromm located health in embracing the freedom won for individuals by capitalism. Paul Tillich was also something of an individualist in so far as he centred his account of psychoanalysis and religion in terms of each individual's finite being or existence. Viktor Frankl too was an individualist in encouraging patients voluntaristically to exert their individual "will to meaning". Melanie Klein's theory is also individualistic in rooting love and hate in individually-given instincts. So too is Marion Milner's recovery of mysticism for psychoanalysis in locating its source in the individual's illusion of oneness with another.

The revolution towards a more intersubjective stance in therapy was first made particularly evident, at least as regards the work of those surveyed in the above chapters, with Winnicott's understanding of therapy. Certainly others before him recognized its interpersonal character. Freud discovered that, to be effective, psychoanalysis must address and put into words the love, and defences against love, awoken by the analyst in the patient. Jung recognized the therapeutic importance of therapists, as well as their patients, being open to being influenced by each other. Simone Weil described the healing of affliction through love of God. So too did Tillich with his account of the healing of self-division, division from others, and from the ground of being, through accepting being accepted by God. Milner too emphasized the importance of psychotherapy and psychoanalysis providing an ambiance in which the patient feels safe to recover oneness with another.

The revolution brought about by Winnicott and others was to emphasize that the illusions, fantasies, and dreams bringing the psyche alive are themselves brought into being not through an individually given will or instinct but through the oneness with us of our mothers in first mothering us. Winnicott emphasized that psychoanalysis and psychotherapy also entails intersubjective oneness of psychoanalysts or psychotherapists with their patients. Only through their putting themselves in their patients' shoes, as Winnicott playfully put it, and as I have more than once reiterated, can patients suffering from false self deadness of their spirit become psychologically more fully alive. He put this symbolically in terms of Christ's Easter Day resurrection.

Bion also contributed toward making psychoanalysts and psychotherapists more aware of the interpersonal and intersubjective character of their work. He did this through emphasizing the importance of the psychoanalyst taking in and containing the ineffable sensory nothingness – O – of the patient's experience, including his experience of the analyst, so as to dream and transform it into a form that can be registered and consciously or unconsciously known. Like Winnicott, Bion also put this in religious terms. He likened the psychoanalyst transforming O to the mystic becoming O, and to Christian Platonism incarnating O in God.

This is hardly consonant with either Judaism or Islam which both forbid any such representation of what is spiritual, holy, or divine. It does, however, lend itself to the notion of God as love. And it is with this intersubjective factor, emphasized by Kristeva, that I ended, and in a sense also began, in telling my book's story largely in terms of the love inspiring some of the major figures contributing to making therapy what it is today. But, as I also said at the outset, quoting Hegel, love has its collisions.

Love's collisions arguably contributed to William James finding himself obstructed from achieving oneness with God. They also arguably contributed to Freud's defensiveness against the counter-transference oneness of psychoanalysts with their patients, and against the oneness with what is outside and beyond us involved in mystical experience. Love's collisions also risked involving Jung in acting out in sex the love evoked in and through his psychoanalytic treatment of Sabina Spielrein. Love can collapse into self-love, as it did in Fromm's account of religion and psychoanalysis. Or it can suffer what Tillich called the sin of division from oneself, others, and the ground of being. We can also lose those we love, as befell Frankl with the concentration camp death of his first wife, Tilly.

Love can also suffer the collisions of persecutory fear, splitting, hateful greed and envy, denial, contempt, and control described by Klein in theorizing the anxieties and defences of paranoid–schizoid and depressive states of mind.

Oneness with another in love can also arouse fears of becoming submerged, swallowed, and destroyed, as described by Milner. We may block off love into a walled-off true self as theorized by Winnicott. Or we may turn the frustration of love into a beta-element thing as conceptualized by Bion. Love can also suffer the annihilation resulting from fusing with another, thereby obliterating recognition of the separation that Kristeva emphasizes is the precondition of love.

This brings me to a problem I raised at the end of my chapter about Kristeva's emphasis on love in bringing together psychoanalysis and religion. It is raised not only by her work but also by that of Winnicott and Bion. For if, as all three say, psychoanalysis entails psychoanalysts imagining themselves into, containing, and transforming the raw data of their patients' experience into fantasy, illusion, and dreams, then this risks mistaking the truth of the patient's experience. There is also the risk of the ineffable, transcendent character of what lies at the heart of psychoanalysis, religion, psychotherapy, and love becoming either the source of dogma, free-for-all relativism, or anything-goes cynicism. This risk can only be circumvented through psychoanalysts and psychotherapists keeping their hunches, interpretations, preconceptions, and so on, open to being tested against whatever subsequently transpires in their interpersonal involvement with their patients. This entails bearing with not knowing, with uncertainty, and oftentimes with silence and emptiness. It entails having the courage not to ward off fear of being overwhelmed by what might emerge in the void through premature formulation. It is precisely this self-same openness to what is happening in, and between, and around us that, as Freud emphasized, is the essence of mental health.

Health entails facing the truth. It is a matter of science. It entails adopting a scientific attitude, equated by Plato with love of wisdom, with love oriented towards discovering what is true. This returns me to the question with which I began. I started with scientific evidence from researchers working for the World Health Organization in Geneva that women's and men's well-being is positively correlated with their spiritual and personal religious belief. I asked what implications this might have for therapy. The answer, it seems, is that therapists must have belief: faith in human nature, according to Winnicott; faith in ultimate reality, according to Bion; faith in love, according to Kristeva.

Therapists, it appears from the work explored in this book's foregoing chapters, must have faith in love of what is true and good, which some equate with God. This entails having faith that the goodness of truth (which can involve what is bad as well as good) can be recovered from unconsciousness through the experiential truth of dreams and illusions, including the illusion of oneness with another as metaphorically or actually divine. That, finally, is what this book has been about.

Index